William Porter

# Diet and Fitness Explained

For Eddie and Elvis

# Contents

1.  Introduction

There are a few points worth covering at the outset.

Firstly, the main purpose of this book is to explain the whole riddle of diet and fitness. Many people find it frustrating that what they enjoy in life is also what is worst for them. The know what food to eat to stay slim and healthy, and what food is bad for them and causes them to be overweight and unhealthy. Wouldn't it be great if you only wanted the healthy food, and had no interest in the unhealthy food? After all, this is what most animals seem able to do. Most species eat what they enjoy, when they want it, they stop when they have had enough and they are generally the perfect size and shape. Some of course have fat on them, but generally this is because they are supposed to have this, for example to keep out the cold.

So why do humans not seem to work in this way? Why are we attracted to food that makes us overweight, that leads to all sorts of health problems, even to an early death? What has gone wrong for us?

It helps to think of it like using a computer. How many times have you been using a computer and become extremely frustrated because it isn't doing what you want it to do? You do something expecting a certain result and not only does the expected result not happen, but something seemingly completely unrelated takes place. I am writing this on Word. Generally it works well, but when I try to number paragraphs the whole thing seems to disintegrate. The numbering will suddenly revert to a completely unrelated and out of sync number, the spacing will change, the indent will suddenly increase or decrease seemingly at random. Have the programmers deliberately put in glitches to make life as difficult as possible? Or is it just that I don't fully understand how it works? Obviously it's the latter. If you don't fully understand something, you run the risk of losing control over it. Would you put a child (or even an adult) with no understanding of how a car works in a car and let them try to drive it? Of course not; if you did, the result would be catastrophic.

Diet and fitness are the same. To get control of it you need to understand it, or more specifically understand how your body and mind works, and how diet and exercise affect it. This is the primary purpose of this book.

Secondly, it is worth mentioning now that I use the word 'diet' in the title, and often in the book itself. To be clear, when I do so I am referring to the food we choose to eat long term on a day to day basis, rather than using it in the context of 'going on a diet', which refers to a short-term restriction on what food we eat.

Thirdly, you may have blanched when I made reference to 'understanding your mind', expecting a book dealing with the power of 'positive thought'. Please rest assured it is nothing so insubstantial. I deal only with well documented, scientific and easily recognisable psychological processes.

Fourthly, it is worth mentioning that I have a rather direct writing style. As one reviewer put it:

'The author is an ex-paratrooper I believe... The military precision in his explanations waste no time by circumventing a subject to fill out prose with empty rhetoric as some other authors do'.

I think this sums things up well. This book is quite short. This is purely because I have quite a direct style and the knack of summarising ideas and concepts in a few words. If I can say something in ten words instead of a hundred words I will do so. This is particularly important given that this isn't a great work of fiction that is designed to take you away to a magical land of your own imagination. If it were then I can see how you would want it to be as long as possible. But it isn't. The point of this book is to assist you towards, hopefully, a better life. If it can do this within an hour instead of ten then it should do so. All books are like a journey; with novels the pleasure is in the journey, not the destination. It's like going on a cruise where the method of travel is the point of the holiday. However, this is not a novel; it is, in essence, a self-help book, and the key with self-help books is very much the destination rather than the journey. To continue with the holiday analogy, it's like taking an uncomfortable plane flight in economy class, surrounded by screaming children and drunken teenagers, to a luxurious holiday destination. You want the journey to be over as quickly as possible so you can get on with the holiday. The worth of this book is not its length but whether it has anything within it that assists you towards improving your life. Please bear in mind that I am not, first and foremost, a writer; I am writing this book because I have information that I believe will be of use to people. I communicate this as best as I am able. This is not going to be the most perfectly polished piece of immaculately crafted literature you will have ever read, but hopefully it will have information that will assist you.

For those familiar with my book on alcohol, there are some small overlaps. Some aspects in particular are directly relevant to both topics (for example the workings of the subconscious, the craving cycle, the effect of drugs on our fitness, and dehydration). I cover them again in this book because it is intended that this book be a complete work on the subject of diet and fitness. So if you have previously read *Alcohol Explained* you can expect some small amount of overlap.

Next, you may find I repeat points. This is not because you have been 'brainwashed' and need 'counter brainwashing' as many writers on this subject say. I have absolutely no interest in repeating points. I say it once and leave it if I can. However, some points are repeated, somethings several times, for one very good reason. Whilst this book breaks down diet and exercise into its constituent parts so we can dissect, analyse and understand each aspect, each individual part is not standalone; it is influenced by the other parts. They all interlink and we experience them all in conjunction with one another. It is impossible to deal properly with each topic without referring it, and cross-referencing it, to the other topics. This not only puts it into context but also explains how it can be influenced by other factors. It is necessary therefore to repeat some ideas and concepts when relating them to other ideas and concepts. I also explain some ideas and concepts several times in different ways to ensure that my meaning is clear. Again, if you catch on the first time and find the repetition annoying then please bear with me, as some people benefit from having things explained several times in different ways.

Next, this book covers new material. There is a lot of it, and much of it is key when looking to understand fully the topic of diet and exercise. However, it is not all new. To clarify, diet and fitness, like the topic of alcohol and addiction, is one of those areas where there is too much information. There are too many ideas, too many opinions, and too much data. What you need to know to understand the topic fully tends to become confused. The key to making sense of it is partly to use some information that has been out there for a while, partly to use information that has been out there for a while but to draw different conclusions to those usually drawn, and partly to incorporate some entirely new ideas and ways of thinking. Think of it as building up a picture: this particular picture is in the form of a jigsaw puzzle of a hundred pieces. However, with this puzzle many of the hundred pieces you actually need are missing, and to make things even more complicated there are an extra thousand pieces that have been mixed in that have nothing to do with the picture we are trying to see. What needs to be done is to firstly extract the relevant pieces from the irreverent pieces and disregard the irrelevant parts. Next, we need to put together what we have. Then we need to fill in the missing parts. Only then can we see things as they actually are. So while there is new information and new ideas in this book, there are also some concepts that have been covered by other writers on this subject previously. I cover them again for the same reason I cover in this book topics I covered in *Alcohol Explained*. It is because it is intended that this book be a complete work on the subject, rather than one that needs to be read in conjunction with others.

Finally, the main problem with writing a book that breaks something down into its constituent parts, each part of which is interrelated with other parts, is that the order is impossible to perfect. Wherever you start you need to relate to topics not yet covered, so there is a lot of 'this is covered in more detail in a later chapter'. I have done the best I can with this and have covered everything in the best order I can, but please bear in mind it is impossible not to refer forwards, particularly in the earlier chapters.

## 2. The Basics

The food we eat contains calories. A calorie is a measure of energy. This energy is needed by us to sustain life. We need energy for our heart to pump, for our lungs to work, and for our organs to function. We also use energy to move; the more we move the more energy we use up.

If we consume more energy than we use up, our body will store it as fat. If we burn up more energy than we consume, our body will use our fat (which is in effect a store of energy) to make up the deficit, and we will lose weight.

These are the basics we need to keep in mind: consume more energy than you burn up and you get fat; burn more energy than you consume and you lose weight. There are an untold number of diets out there advocating weird and wonderful ways to lose weight, but this is the one inescapable fact; it is simple physics. It doesn't matter if you think you have a slow metabolism, a genetic disposition to carry more fat, an inability to burn off fat, or are too old to lose weight. Your body cannot make something out of nothing. If you consume 2,000 calories and burn off 2,500, you will lose weight.

This may seem too obvious to need to state, but it is often lost in these complicated and convoluted diets of having to eat this or not being able to eat that, or you can only eat a certain type of food with another certain type or at a certain time, or people believing that there is something genetically different about them, or that you can enter 'famine mode' and actually gain fat the less you eat as your body becomes more inclined to store energy as fat, or that weight becomes harder to lose as you get older, etc. The simple fact is that if you consume more energy or calories than you use, you will gain weight (or more specifically fat) and if you burn off more than you consume, you will lose weight.

At its simplest, if you want to lose weight you need to burn off more energy than you consume. So far so good. But how do you do this? Well, there are only three ways. Firstly, you can consume fewer calories. Secondly, you can exercise more. Thirdly, you can do both.

So if it is this straightforward, why is it so hard to lose weight? Why are so many people obese? Why is there such an obesity epidemic in the

14

Western world? The answer to this is also simple: hunger. If you suddenly start eating less, you get hungry. Exercising may initially seem like an ideal solution as you should be able to eat the same, start exercising, and lose weight. Unfortunately it doesn't work this way, because when you exercise you just get hungrier. Your body triggers feelings of hunger in many situations, one of which is when you get low on readily available energy (i.e. energy from food rather than energy stored as fat). Your body stores excess energy as fat in case food becomes scarce, and it doesn't want to use this backup store unless it has to, so you can have huge amounts of excess energy stored as fat but still feel hungry because your body wants to avoid using the fat stores unless it has to.

So although exercise may seem like a good way to lose weight as you should be able to eat the same amount of food but burn off more and thus lose weight, it doesn't work this way because exercise makes you hungry so you just end up eating more. The usual recommendation to maintain weight is 2,000 calories a day for females and 2,500 calories a day for males. Let's say you are consuming 3,000 calories a day and doing no exercise and getting fat. If you then start exercising and burn off 4,000 calories a day you won't automatically lose weight because those 3,000 calories will no longer satisfy you – you will still be hungry after them. So you still end up finding yourself up against hunger.

All living creatures have hunger as a driving force to keep them alive. It is an extremely powerful force; hunger can drive people to rob, to steal and to kill. The reason dieting is so difficult is that it is essentially a battle with hunger, that overwhelming and very powerful force. Whatever the diet, whatever the exercise routine, it all comes down to a battle with hunger.

So now we have the basics in place. They may seem very simple and very self-explanatory, but it is worth running through them and highlighting them, as dieting is one of the many things in life where the problem is not lack of information, but quite the opposite: there is too much information, too many ideas and too many competing theories. It has become overcomplicated and it is useful sometimes to go back to the basics. One of the keys to understanding it is to keep in mind the basic irrefutable facts, focus in on the key points and ignore the irrelevant or ancillary points. The only way to lose weight is to burn off more energy than you consume, but the problem is that when you start to do this, you start to feel hungry.

So the very first thing we need to do if we want to lose weight is to understand hunger by dissecting it, breaking it down into its constituent parts, and analysing it so we can understand this barrier that stops us from losing weight. However, before we do this, it helps to have a basic understanding of how our digestive system works.

3.  Our Digestive System

There has been an advertising campaign in the UK stating that obesity is the second highest cause of preventable cancer after smoking. I do not agree with this. Obesity isn't a cause of cancer, it is a symptom of overeating, and in particular eating the wrong food. Cancer is also a symptom of the same thing. It is overeating and eating the wrong type of food that is the problem, and a problem that causes both obesity and cancer.

We seem to have this rather strange view of overeating – we know it causes us to become overweight and can cause health problems (like diabetes and cancer), but other than this we don't see any downside to it. The actual immediate negative impact is largely ignored.

In fact, digestion itself takes a huge amount of effort. How much of an effort depends on the food we eat. Our bodies find it easiest to process liquids rather than solids, so food with a high water content (such as fruit and vegetables) is far easier to digest. I deal in detail with what food we should be eating later on in this book, but for now let's consider digestion and in particular the effort involved in digesting food.

Once in the stomach, chewed food has to be churned in order to mix it with various digestive enzymes. This churning process is hard work, and to undertake it the body redirects a large portion of the blood supply from the muscles in the extremities to the stomach and intestines. This is why we often feel tired or drained, and why it is not unusual to sleep, after eating a large meal.

After the stomach is through churning, the partially digested food is moved into the small intestine, where it is mixed with more digestive juices. Some nutrients are absorbed at this stage, then the remainder is passed into the large intestine. There, water and the vital mineral salts dissolved in that water are extracted and absorbed into the blood stream through thin permeable membranes. The final residue is squeezed along the length of the large intestines and passes out of the body.

The process by which food moves through your digestive tract is known as peristalsis. The organs of your digestive system contain a layer of muscle that enables their walls to move. The muscle behind the food contracts and squeezes the food forward, while the muscle in front of the food relaxes to allow the food to move. The total distance this food has to move is 30 feet. There is 30 feet of digestive tract for it to cover, every inch of which it has to be pushed through by the digestive muscles.

If the food we are eating is difficult to digest then all of this takes a huge amount of effort and while it is taking place we feel drained and tired. As you can imagine, although it leaves us feeling tired and we are tempted to sleep, the sleep we get when digesting food is not good quality sleep. Digestion not only takes a huge amount of energy, it also creates a huge amount of movement and a frenzy of activity. This internal churning, movement and activity disturbs our sleep with the result that we tend to need to sleep longer and feel less refreshed when we wake up. Also, as any physicist will tell you, all energy ultimately ends up as heat energy, so the process of digestion tends to make us warm, which is another thing that disturbs sleep. Lots of the drugs we take on a regular basis tend to disturb our sleep (this is dealt with in more detail in a later chapter), but if you seem to be tired all the time, and find you wake up at night hot and uncomfortable, you may find changing your eating habits helps. Needless to say, smaller, lighter meals (and by lighter I mean a greater proportion of easily digestible food, or food with a high water content like fruit and vegetables) is far less effort for our bodies to digest, and making sure you have your last meal several hours before going to bed also helps.

So overeating and bad diet doesn't just cause us long terms problems like cancer and obesity, it also causes us short terms problems like lethargy and sleep disturbance (particularly if you, like many people, tend to eat a lot in the evening before going to bed). This is a less well known but (for me at least) a far more important impact of overeating and bad diet. Let me be clear on this point: I am not saying that cancer and obesity is worse than lethargy and disturbed sleep, but for me the short-term implications always weigh more heavily than the long-term implications. Everyone dies, and what happens to me in 20 or 30 years simply causes less concern for me than what happens to me today and tomorrow. This may seem incredibly short sighted and irresponsible of me, and maybe it is, but it is what it is. If you offer me a pleasure today but tell me it may have a detrimental effect in 30 years, I'll take the pleasure and worry about it in 20 or 30 years' time. But if that pleasure is fleeting and lasts only for a few seconds, and the detriment will be felt a few minutes after that, and will last all night and into the following day, AND will impact me in 20 or 30 years then there's no contest. I'll forgo the pleasure and not worry in the least about it.

Another point to bear in mind with indigestible food like pizza, burgers, red meat and processed foods like pasta and bread is that because your body cannot easily digest it, the muscles of the digestive system have to work extremely hard to process it. This requires energy: energy that your body is struggling to extract from the rubbish you have just eaten. It needs an immediate, readily available and readily absorbable hit of energy, so you will crave something sweet, something with refined sugar. This is why if you overeat savoury food you can be so full you can scarcely move, be so full you feel physically sick, but still crave something sweet. It's the body crying out for readily available energy. This is why you often crave something sweet after a large, processed food-based meal.

The knock-on effect of this is that your body cannot dedicate enough energy to processing the rubbish you've eaten, and you will feel tired and lethargic as your body struggles to get to grips with it, but there is nothing it can really do. It needs to focus far more of your body's resources to doing this. So how does it do this? It waits until you are asleep, then it really gets to work on it. This is why so many people evacuate their bowels first thing in the morning; it is because their body has worked on the food overnight. The problem with this is not only the effect on sleep, which we have already covered, but also that your body is then extracting the vast majority of the huge number of empty calories from what you have eaten whilst you are asleep. As you are not actively moving at this time, these calories are far more likely to be stored as fat. Contrast this with fruit and vegetables, which are far easier to digest and have readily available energy, but energy that is released slowly so you can actually use it.

This is why you have these well documented cases of people who consume way over their recommended daily intake of calories in fresh fruit and vegetables, and yet are slim and healthy looking, whereas people who consume far less actual calories in the form or processed, nutrient sparse, low fibre and low water content food will pile on the weight.

This is a key point that is worth keeping at the forefront of your mind, because it can be confusing. There is all the difference in the world between the 'slow release' and 'indigestible'. 'Slow Release' means the energy is absorbed slowly so we don't get the spikes and lows or hunger straight after (again this is dealt with in a later chapter). Slow release energy is found in fresh fruit, vegetables, nuts, beans, rice, seeds, oats, legumes etc. It is very easy for your body to digest this sort of food (indeed it is precisely what your body is best able to process), it is just that the energy boost from it is gradual and long lasting. 'Indigestible' means your body struggles to digest it. We are often told that 'slow release' is best, and this is correct, but then we assume (understandably) that something that is difficult to digest must also be slow release (after all, it must take far longer for the body to extract the energy from it) and we also assume that if it's in us longer then it leaves us feeling fuller for longer. This makes sense until we start to understand that 'feeling full' doesn't always mean 'not feeling hungry' or 'not wanting to eat food'. Indeed, eating the wrong food can leave you feeling bloated and hungry at the same time (again this is covered in more detail later in the book).

This is why fasting has such well documented health benefits. There have been numerous studies on the effects of fasting and there is a clear connection between fasting and improved immunity, reduced inflammation, reduced cancer incident, reduced likelihood of diabetes, reduced heart disease and increased energy levels. There are lots of ways people practise fasting, from methods that require you to eat very little for one or two days a week, to systems that require periods each day consuming nothing. The reason that fasting is so beneficial is that digestion is an onerous process and giving your body a break gives it some time to recuperate, and also to sleep properly.

We tend to think that eating gives us energy, and it does, but only if we are eating the right food in the right amounts. If you are eating food that is difficult to digest, and eating too much of it, you are going to find your energy levels are constantly low due to the energy being diverted, the indigestion and the disturbed sleep. This type of food is primarily digested at night when it is far more likely to be stored as fat. This is why, although it may seem counterintuitive, cutting back on food and eating lighter food actually leaves you feeling more energetic.

Obviously if you wish to experiment with different types of fasting than you can do so; the purpose of this book is not to provide rules you have to obey, but to explain the basics so you can do what is best for you. The point I wish to make here is not whether to fast or not fast, but merely to explain how and why eating less, and eating lighter, leaves you feeling more energetic and healthier generally. This has an immediate, very positive impact, and a long-term impact, on your day to day life, and greatly outbalances the frustrating and dubious 'pleasure' of overeating and poor diet.

When we think of eating / not eating, we tend of think very simply along the lines of eating being good, and not eating leading to starvation and being bad. We need to stop thinking along these lines. How many people do you know who have starved to death? How many people do you know who are overweight? The diet-associated problems we encounter in the Western world aren't generally deficiencies, but excesses.

Now that we have a basic understanding of how our digestive system works, we can dissect and understand the phenomenon of hunger (i.e. a desire to eat).

4.  Hunger – Taste

One of the obvious aspects of 'hunger' (or a desire to eat something) is taste. If something tastes good, we enjoy eating it. But actually it's not as simple as this. Think of something you really enjoy eating. If you ate it to excess all day every day you'd soon become sick of it, and the smell and taste of it would repulse you. The smell and taste hasn't changed, but its effect on you has.

In fact, hunger and what food we choose is a very convoluted process. Humans (and in fact all animals) can eat many things, some good for them, some less good for them, some actively poisonous to them. To a certain degree we have an inbuilt, instinctive ability to determine the difference between food and poison; things that are good for us taste good, things that are bad for us don't. But as anyone knows who enjoys alcoholic drinks, cigarettes, coffee, burgers, chocolate or any other of the (seemingly) several billion things that taste good but are bad for you, things aren't this simple.

Firstly, we humans do tend to mess around with things. We're always trying to improve things but in doing so we often we just make things worse for ourselves. For example, fruit contains sugar; it is generally sweet. Fruit is good for us, so we have a preprogrammed taste for sweet things to encourage us to eat fruit. But the problem is we take the sugar out of the fruit, refine it, remove all the vitamins and minerals, and consume it in far greater concentrations than our bodies are designed to deal with. We get all the calories without any of the associated nutrition. We then add it to things that might otherwise taste vile (i.e. they are bad for us) to make them taste good (like coffee, cocoa, alcohol etc.). This causes all kinds of problems, including not only obesity but also diabetes and high blood pressure.

Secondly, and perhaps more importantly, humans and all animals have the ability to adapt their diet in times of need. Whilst living creatures do have an innate or pre-existing ability to differentiate between poison and food through smell and taste (i.e. one that is in their genes), they also have the ability to adapt it. When we are drained, tired, hungry, etc. eating will make us feel better, both physically and mentally. So if we consume something that we wouldn't necessarily think of as food, or something that tastes or smells offensive, and we feel immediately better after we consume it (or if it relieves hunger or tiredness), and providing it doesn't make us immediately ill, on a subconscious level the brain will conclude that what we immediately identified as poison actually had some form of nutritional benefit, i.e. that it is 'food' rather than 'poison', and as it didn't seem to harm us we can continue to consume it. As such, over time, we will cease to be repulsed by the smell and taste of it; instead, we will start to find it appetising and will start to hunger for it. In this way if a living creature's food source becomes scarce or disappears, they will be able to adapt to other food types through trial and error. Again, from an evolutionary point of view this makes sense; most if not all species encounter a shortage of food at some point. If they simply stopped eating when food ran out then the species would die out. They have to be able to experiment with new food sources and to adapt. This is a key element of survival. Not many living creatures on the planet have such a reliable food source that they never have the need to adapt to an alternative during leaner times.

As a child I found the smell of Stilton (a very mature blue cheese) repugnant. I remember seeing my father eat it and wondering how anyone could want to eat something so vile. However, I used to have a very watered-down version of it by having soup with a small amount of it crumbled in. I also kept trying it on the odd occasion. Now I eat it quite happily – in fact, I 'like' the flavour of it. The smell and taste remain the same, they haven't changed, it is just that on a subconscious level my body and brain has realised that it doesn't make me physically ill and it also relieves hunger. Thus have I become able to eat it, and even, eventually, to enjoy it. You only have to look at the different cuisines and diets being consumed by human beings the world over to note this phenomenon. Inuits will happily eat and enjoy raw, frozen whale meat; the Mongols used to drink blood direct from cuts on their horses' necks and Aborigines will eat the witchetty grub, which is a large maggot. These are obviously extreme examples, but they highlight how humans can eat and 'enjoy' a huge range of food. Inuits, Mongols and Aborigines are not born with a genetic difference that causes them to enjoy these types of food, they are simply brought up eating them.

This phenomenon also has a direct impact on drug addiction. A drug can make us feel immediately better, not because it has nutritional benefit, but because it interferes with our chemical functioning such that we feel better even though the actual physical effect is a negative one. In this way we can learn to want, or to hunger for, any drug we take regularly.

Although living things can adapt to a new diet in times of need, there is an ingrained reluctance to do so, and it is usually hunger that drives a species to it. When we have a tried and tested food source we tend to stick to it. Again I think this is a fairly natural tendency. After all, as far as your survival mechanism is concerned, if you have tried something and found it to be nutritional and not poisonous, why would you try something else, which may actually be poisonous? After all, not all poisons taste bad. So there is a pronounced tendency to stick with and favour the food we eat regularly. Think of young children: they tend to be very unadventurous with their food. They find something they like and never want to eat anything else.

So where do we get to if we consider these two aspects (the ability to adapt our diet and our inherent reluctance to do so) together? Firstly, we need to bear in mind that the food we currently 'enjoy' may not be the most beneficial for us. In fact, it may not even be the food we would enjoy the most if we gave other foods a fair chance. Secondly, healthy food isn't necessarily food we won't enjoy.

The point to take away from this chapter is that we can change the food we 'like'. It takes a bit of time, and a bit of effort, but it can be done gradually and in time we can change our eating habits long term. We will deal later on with what foods we ought to cut back on and what foods we need to eat more of from a diet and fitness point of view, but for now all we need to do is understand is that it is entirely possible to change what we 'enjoy'.

## 5.   Hunger – The Subconscious

The term 'subconscious' is used in a myriad of different ways to cover an untold number of different processes; it is almost a catch-all for anything we do that we don't fully understand. When I use the term, I am referring to the process by which certain actions can become automated if they are repeated regularly and seem to confer a benefit. Ever had a power cut and found yourself turning on light switches every time you went into a dark room even though you knew there was no electricity? Ever found your left leg tensing when you are in the passenger seat of a car and the driver is driving too fast? Ever found yourself punching in your old password automatically when logging on to your computer after a password change? If you do something regularly and it confers an apparent benefit, that behaviour will be triggered 'subconsciously' (i.e. without you having to make a conscious decision to do it) when the apparent benefit is required. So walk into a dark room, reach for the light switch, turn your computer on and punch in the password, extend your left leg to slow down a car, eat something if you are feeling a bit low and need a boost.

If you do something and it makes you feel good in certain situations or alleviates negative feelings, it will start to impact your subconscious, so that whenever you are in need of a boost, or need to alleviate a negative feeling (such as loneliness, anger, depression, etc.), your subconscious will trigger the thought of whatever it is you have become conditioned to reach for.

The subconscious is an amazing thing – it automates actions that we would otherwise have to think about consciously, saving precious seconds in an emergency situation, freeing up your mind to concentrate on other things. However, although it is an amazing thing on one level, on another level it is incredibly stupid. It works only on immediate cause and effect, and has no ability to rationalise beyond this. So if you are a driver and are in a car where the driver is leaving braking too late, your left leg will be tensing. Your subconscious will be doing this because throughout your life as a driver it will have absorbed the message that pressing down on your left leg will slow down a vehicle. It won't be able to reason that in the current circumstances you are in fact in the passenger seat with no brake pedal, it is literally just an instinctive reaction based on previous cause and effect.

Although this subconscious reaction is a large part of our lives, it tends to go unnoticed. We take it for granted. However, one area where it does feature quite prominently is in the area of drug addiction. For example, cigarettes contain nicotine, which is a stimulant, so when you smoke a cigarette you feel more alert mentally than you did previously. Alcohol is an anaesthetic and a depressant (by which I mean it inhibits or depresses nerve activity) and so it depresses feelings of tiredness, anxiety, nervousness, depression, etc. Again, the subconscious simply links cause with immediate effect, so it will associate smoking with enhanced alertness and cause you to keep reaching for a cigarette. It will not factor into its reasoning the cancer, heart disease etc., and even more importantly it will be unable to realise that as the brain starts to anticipate the regular introduction of an external stimulant, it will cease releasing its own internal and naturally occurring stimulants, so you then need to smoke a cigarette to feel normal. The position is then worsened even further as the erosion of fitness that accompanies any long-term intake of a drug (which I deal with in more detail in a later chapter) and the clogging up of the respiratory system actually leaves you, within a very short space of time, less alert and awake even while smoking the cigarette compared to had you never smoked in the first place. However, all the subconscious knows is that you smoke a cigarette and get an immediate short-term boost, so it keeps prompting you to reach for one. Again, with alcohol, the subconscious only links the consuming of the drink with the immediate anaesthetising effect – it cannot factor in the intoxication, the hangover and all the other negatives associated with drinking.

You can probably already start to see how the subconscious can impact our diet. When you are tired and hungry and even aching after vigorous exercise or work, eating can make you feel considerably better. It can relieve the hunger, give you some energy, and greatly improve how you feel. The subconscious very quickly links the cause (eating) to the effect (feeling better) and you can soon find yourself reaching for something to eat every time you feel in need of a boost. Again, the subconscious won't be able to differentiate between different types of 'needing a boost'. For example, if you are feeling under 100% because you are hungry and need nutrients, then eating will indeed give you a boost. But if you don't need energy or nutrients, and are feeling low not because of something physical, but something mental (like loneliness, low self-esteem, anxiety, etc.), eating won't do anything for you at all, other than leave you feeling uncomfortably full and guilty, which in actuality will leave you feeling worse off. However, as far as your subconscious reasoning goes it is simple: feel low, reach for something to eat.

So these subconscious triggers can trigger 'hunger', or a desire to eat. They create a marked tendency to reach for food every time we are feeling low, but in fact there are two other aspects of 'hunger' which exacerbate the impact eating has on our subconscious. We will cover these in the next two chapters.

## 6.   Hunger – Dopamine and the Physiological Side of Eating

Dopamine is a chemical that makes us feel good. It is naturally occurring in humans and other animals. It is released when we do things that are beneficial for 'us' personally, or 'us' as a species. It is an integral part of survival. By making humans and animals feel good when they eat, reproduce, exercise etc. you create a species that naturally does things to survive and multiply. Whether you believe that humans were created by God or by a process of natural selection is neither here nor there. The fact is that it exists, and it motivates us to act in certain ways.

When you eat, you receive a burst of dopamine and this makes you feel better than you did before you ate. As you can probably work out for yourself, this will have a direct impact on your subconscious. Your subconscious will start to associate eating with the dopamine boost and the (minor) relief of stress, anger, depression, unhappiness, loneliness, etc.

This is why for many people whenever they suffer a setback, be it an argument, a feeling of low self-esteem, loneliness, anything in fact that makes them feel a bit low, the instinctive thought enters their mind to eat something. For some people it might be to have a cigarette, or a drink, but for some of us it is to have something to eat.

Now the problem is of course that overeating causes its own problems, one of which is to make us fat. And of course, being fat makes most people feel low. They feel ugly and it gives them low self-esteem. Let me be perfectly clear on this point, I am not saying being overweight does make you unattractive or ugly, but there is absolutely no doubt that it makes many people feel unattractive or ugly. It makes them feel bad. And this of course triggers the thought of eating, and so the problem deteriorates. It is a vicious circle, and it becomes progressively worse as things progress.

The problem is that you only get the dopamine boost when you are hungry and have something nutritious to eat. If you aren't hungry, if your digestive system is already fully engaged dealing with food and you have no caloric shortage, eating more won't give you a dopamine boost but it will leave you feeling uncomfortably full, guilty and frustrated. However, your subconscious won't know this – all it knows is that when you are feeling low, eating can make you feel better, so it keeps you reaching for something to eat.

Some people reading this may not be in this position. They may not want to eat every time they need a boost. They may use other methods to get that boost when they feel low, such as smoking or drinking or having a cup of tea or coffee. However, all of these things create their own, similar, vicious circles which also lead to weight gain. The effect of these crutches we use on weight are dealt with in a later chapter.

So a small, healthy meal makes you feel good. You associate eating with feeling good. If you feel bad, you eat. But whilst eating a small amount until you feel full will make you feel better, eating more will make you feel uncomfortable, frustrated and bad tempered. You don't get more endorphins for eating more than your fill but your subconscious doesn't know this. It just associates eating with feeling good. If you are miserable and you eat when you are genuinely hungry, you will get a dopamine boost. But when you are full you will still be miserable (albeit maybe marginally less miserable then you were before). However, because you are still miserable your subconscious will continue to trigger the thought of eating more to relieve the misery.

This is a key point to bear in mind. Eating and satisfying a genuine hunger will be enjoyable and give you a boost; continuing to eat after you have satisfied this hunger will bring you increasingly down the more you over eat.

So a desire to get a boost can also trigger a desire to eat, but we need to be very careful as this particular form of 'hunger' is often false, and eating won't bring about the desired result.

## 7.  Hunger – the Ups and Downs of Refined Sugar

Imagine if you took something healthy, like an apple or spinach or broccoli, and removed one specific nutrient from it, and concentrated it a thousandfold and started eating it eight or nine times a day. I don't think it would be any great stretch of the imagination to think that our bodies might be unable to cope with this, having never before had to deal with it. This is not far off what we do with sugar. But the ridiculous thing is that we then identify sugar as a problem and seek to avoid any food with it in, even if it is naturally occurring. Your body is designed to cope with naturally occurring sugars, like those in fruit. It's only when we concentrate and refine it and eat too much of it that it causes us problems like obesity and diabetes.

I think everyone is aware that there are substantial arguments to suggest that refined sugar is bad for you. The confusing part is that naturally occurring sugar is fine, so often people think that refined sugar is also ok as long as you have it in small doses like in fruit; as long as you are careful with it and don't go mad, it is fine. After all, everyone says fruit is good for you, and fruit contains sugar, so sugar can't be bad for you in and of itself. In fact this isn't the case: refined sugar is chemically different from naturally occurring sugar, and how our body reacts to refined sugars and natural sugars is very different. Really, refined sugar and natural sugar should have completely different names, as the ways they affect us are very different.

I don't think it is necessary to plunge deep into the chemical physiological processes of sugar absorption, but having said this, a basic understanding does assist.

When sugar enters the bloodstream, the body releases insulin. Insulin allows the organs, muscles and nerve cells of the body to absorb the sugar and use it.

So here you have a very (very) basic explanation of sugar and insulin. You eat something with sugar, it ends up in the blood stream, insulin is released, and the insulin is the method by which the sugar is removed from the blood and is utilised by the parts of the body that need it.

The difference between natural sugar and refined sugar is that the refined sugar enters the blood stream far faster than the natural sugar, indeed far faster than is natural and far faster than our body is able to deal with. This huge surge in blood sugar causes the body to release a surge of insulin to regulate the blood sugar, the blood sugar is then very quickly dealt with, which leaves too little blood sugar, causing you to feel drained and tired and in need of another sugar rush.

It helps sometimes to think of it in terms of numbers just for illustrative purposes. Let's compare what happens if you consume five points of natural sugar, compared to five points of refined sugar.

Let's assume you eat five points of natural sugar, and it enters your bloodstream at a rate of one point of sugar every ten minutes (so the total amount of sugar entering the bloodstream will be a steady flow over 50 minutes). As soon as the first point of sugar reaches your bloodstream, your body will sense the sugar and release exactly the right amount of insulin to deal with the amount of sugar over the next 50 minutes. How does it know how much sugar will be entering the blood stream? Because since the very dawn of the human race all sugars we have consumed are

44

naturally occurring sugars, they are the only kind our bodies know (refined sugars may have been around for a few years now, but in evolutionary terms they have scarcely been around for a millisecond). The body knows that what enters in the first ten minutes will be a steady flow over the next 50 minutes. So it will release one point of insulin, which will remain in the blood for the next 50 minutes, and that insulin will be processing one point of sugar every ten minutes.

So everything is all nice and easy and a perfect balance.

However, let's now eat five points of refined sugar. Because of its chemical composition all five points are released into the bloodstream at once, and your body therefore releases five points of insulin (don't forget your body isn't designed to deal with refined sugar, it is specifically designed only for naturally occurring sugars). These five points of insulin will remove five points of sugar from your blood every ten minutes for 50 minutes. The first ten minutes is fine, the blood sugar level is balanced, but after that there is no additional sugar entering the bloodstream, which there would be if you had eaten naturally occurring sugar which takes far longer to enter the bloodstream. What happens after this first ten minutes, however, is that the insulin continues to process sugar in the blood, but no additional sugar is entering the blood stream, with the result that your blood sugar level starts to drop too low.

This is essentially the sugar crash we have all heard about (and most likely experienced). The key point to note is that it ends up with a sugar/insulin imbalance, with too much insulin and not enough sugar. So what's the quickest and easiest remedy? More refined sugar of course. So what you ultimately end up with is refined sugar causing an internal imbalance which more sugar will rectify. This is in fact the basis of all drug addiction (with a chemical causing a problem which more of the same chemical will rectify). This is why people compare consumption of refined sugar to drug addiction.

Again, and as with dopamine, if we then factor in the subconscious we can see how the problem starts to increase dramatically. As we have dealt with previously, the subconscious only links cause with immediate effect, i.e. refined sugar consumption with a boost. This boost is even more noticeable if you are suffering from the 'crash' (the low blood sugar) caused by the previous spike in refined sugar. The only conclusion your subconscious draws is simple: consumption of refined sugar = good! As with drug addiction, the subconscious is unable to appreciate that the 'boost' that is received by the consuming of the sugar (or drug) is actually simply to relieve a problem (or imbalance) that was caused by consuming that sugar (or drug) in the first place.

The problem with refined sugar is further exacerbated because, as we know, the subconscious links cause to effect. How quickly it links these depends on three elements. How noticeable the cause is, how noticeable the effect is, and the amount of time between the two. If the cause is easily identifiable, and the effect is equally easily identifiable, and the time between the two is shorter instead of longer, the subconscious will link the cause with the effect far quicker.

To go back to our example, if you eat something with natural sugar (the cause) then the effect is both (relatively) slow to be felt (as it takes longer for the natural sugar to enter the bloodstream) and less noticeable as the boost from the natural sugar intake is more gradual. Compare this to eating something high in refined sugar in which the effect is both far quicker and far more noticeable (as it is far less of a gradual process). In this instance, the subconscious will link the cause and effect of the refined sugar far quicker and far more effectively than the naturally occurring sugar.

This is another key point to lodge very firmly in your mind: the sugar boost from naturally occurring sugar fruit is no less than the sugar boost from refined sugar, it is just that the refined sugar boost is more immediate and noticeable. So not only do you gain absolutely nothing from eating refined sugar as opposed to naturally occurring sugar, but you also cause yourself considerable health problems, one of which is diabetes.

There are two types of diabetes. Type 2 is the one linked to excess sugar consumption. Essentially, what happens is that the constant high levels of refined sugar lead to consistently high amounts of insulin, which in turn lead to the body's cells becoming resistant to insulin, which in turn leads to the body being unable to regulate blood sugar. This then results in the blood sugar level becoming too high and not enough sugar being utilised by the organs, muscles and nerve cells.

So now we've looked at some physiological processes, and the automated reactions of the subconscious mind. Next we will see what happens in our conscious mind when we start craving certain foods.

8. Hunger – Craving

Cravings are when we become fixated on the thought of something, when we fantasise about it and obsess over it and can think of nothing else. It can be triggered by hunger (either hunger due to lack of available energy or due to a lack of a particular nutrient), and it can also be triggered by the subconscious. So you may feel a hunger pang, or feel tired, or low, and your subconscious will trigger the immediate, knee jerk reaction: to reach for something to eat. This will put the thought of food well and truly in your conscious mind. However, you can crave something without any associated physical or subconscious trigger, and it can even exist when we are so full we are actively uncomfortable.

It is useful to think of craving as a cycle, as it is something that goes around and around and becomes increasingly potent as it does so. Let's run through the mental processes involved so we can dissect and understand the craving cycle.

Firstly, there will be something to set off the craving. It may be something physical such as genuine hunger, or thirst, or withdrawal from a drug, or feeling unhappy or tired or depressed. This may be a feeling that you are consciously aware of, so you may feel genuine hunger and think about eating something. However, it may be something that you are not consciously aware of, but that your subconscious picks up on, so the thought of eating enters your conscious mind this way. It may be neither of these things – you may just be walking down the street and pass McDonalds, or see an advert for a soft drink, or see someone eating or drinking something and think you might like to eat it yourself. However it enters your mind, you are now consciously thinking about eating something.

If you start to fantasise about how great it would be to eat or drink whatever it is you are thinking about, and if you start to obsess about it, you will know no peace until you have it. It will occupy your mind to the exclusion of all else. If you are at work, you won't be able to concentrate on your job. If you are out socialising or otherwise (supposedly) enjoying yourself, you will no longer be enjoying what you are doing because you will be too busy wanting something.

One point to note here is that a large part of craving is fantasising. Fantasising is exactly that: it is a FANTASY. It is not reality. When we fantasise about something, we look only at the positive, not the negative – the negative gets entirely ignored. Indeed, even the supposed good gets greatly exaggerated and bears little or no resemblance to reality. How many times have you really wanted to eat something, but then found it doesn't even remotely meet your expectations? This is because what you were thinking about when you were anticipating it was a fantasy – the reality is very different.

Turning back now to the craving process, and assuming you haven't yet given in to it, you are now miserable and you are not enjoying whatever it is you are doing, or concentrating on whatever it is you are supposed to be working on. You can't concentrate on anything other than the object of your craving. At this point the object of your craving isn't really the main issue; the main issue is you are now in a sort of self-imposed tantrum. The craving will continue until, ultimately, you either give in or the situation or day ends.

If you give in then, having ended the craving spiral, you can get on with whatever it was you were supposed to be doing, either working or enjoying yourself or whatever. Of course, as soon as you give in and have it, you immediately end the misery of the craving, so having that item you were craving becomes the difference between being miserable and not being miserable, or if you were otherwise doing something you were enjoying, misery or happiness. It is not the item itself that has caused that jump from misery to joy, it has simply caused a craving process (which makes us decidedly miserable) and then ended the same process.

However, if you don't give in then the whole event is a write off – it is ruined because you couldn't think of anything else other than the object of your craving. All you will remember is that you were miserable because you couldn't have whatever it was you wanted, and the next time you are in that same (or a similar) situation the craving will be that much more potent because you will know from personal experience that you couldn't enjoy yourself without whatever it was you wanted.

The trouble is that we then start to instinctively know that when we start to crave something we are in for a rough ride, and so often (quite understandably) give up on it almost immediately. A part of you knows, when you get home from a grim day at work and plonk yourself down in front of the TV and then remember that chocolate bar in the cupboard, that you won't know a moment's peace until you have it, and that your precious and all too short evening will be ruined until you give in and go and get it. So why waste the time over it? Just get it down your neck as soon as possible to get it out of the way, then you can relax and enjoy your evening.

The problem is that the craving wins either way. If you resist it then you ruin the event or occasion or whatever, so next time the craving is even stronger; and if you give in then you prove to yourself that that item was the difference between misery and joy, so next time you crave it all the more fully because you are craving not just the item but the relief you have proven to yourself that having that item brings.

As you can see, a craving can be very overpowering, and seems to get the upper hand no matter what you do. However, craving is something that takes place purely in the conscious mind, and therefore it is within our control whether to crave or not. Many people struggle with the concept that craving is controllable, mainly because cravings create a cycle that becomes progressively worse, and the only way out seems to be to either suffer it or give in to it. However, there are ways to short circuit the craving cycle without giving in to it and I deal with these in a later chapter. For now let's turn to the final part of what makes up 'hunger'.

## 9. Hunger – Lack of Available Energy and Lack of Nutrients

We've already touched on how hunger is triggered by a lack of readily available energy or calories, but hunger is also triggered by lack of nutrients (i.e. vitamins and minerals that our bodies need to survive and thrive).

Again, if you think about it, this is just common sense. Hunger causes us to eat, but eating doesn't just provide us with calories, it also (if we are eating nutritious food) provides us with vitamins and minerals. So your body won't just trigger hunger when you are low on calories, it will also trigger it if you are low on a particular nutrient.

Vitamins are organic compounds that the body needs in small quantities to function. These are the nutrients that, for the most part, our body does not produce. When these nutrients start to get low, you will start to feel hungrier and you will start to want food that is high in whatever nutrient you are lacking.

Do you like orange, lemon or blackcurrant drinks? Why do you think this is? Because orange, lemon and blackcurrant contain vitamin C, which your body needs, if you start getting low on it your body will trigger a feeling of hunger, and you will start to want something that is high in vitamin C. The problem is, as we've touched on previously, that humans tend to interfere with natural food. Let's say you are getting low on vitamin C and so you are feeling hungry and you buy a burger and fizzy orange drink. The drink will taste wonderful, and the reason it will taste so wonderful is that is tastes of orange and your body therefore thinks it is high in vitamin C. The problem is that there is no vitamin C in it, it only tastes like orange because it has refined sugar in it along with a chemical to make it taste like orange. You've had the calories from the drink, and the calories from the burger which you didn't need, and you've obtained no vitamin C at all (which was what triggered hunger in the first place). As you haven't got the vitamin C you need you still have a feeling of hunger, but now this is accompanied with a feeling of being full. This is one of the most unpleasant and frustrating things about our Western diet: we can actually be hungry and unpleasantly full at one and the same time. Compare this to feeling fit and energetic and well rested. A healthy and sensible diet isn't about wanting to look better or live longer, it is about huge improvements to your quality of life.

I read an article recently that opined that humans do not need to eat fruit and vegetables as they can obtain all the vitamins and minerals they need from multivitamins and supplements. There are several problems with this. Firstly, the vitamins and nutrients in multivitamins and supplements are often synthetic and there is a body of opinion that suggests that these synthetic versions cannot be absorbed and/or utilised in the same way as naturally occurring vitamins can. Secondly, they are often present in greater concentrations than occur naturally and this can cause its own problems. Thirdly, the benefit of having a diet high in fruit and vegetables is only partly due to the nutrients they provide; in fact, the more immediate benefit of this is that fruit and vegetables have a much higher water content and are therefore far easier for the body to digest. Finally, not all vitamins have been discovered and categorised, so limiting yourself to vitamin tablets may end up with you missing out on certain vitamins or nutrients that you may actually need.

Whether your goal is to lose weight or live a better quality of life, you cannot do this without getting the vitamins and minerals you need, because if you are low on vitamins and minerals you will be constantly hungry. This hunger will be like a dripping tap – it will push you and push you and push you and eventually you will eat, but if you are eating the wrong food you will still not get the nutrients you need and you will still be hungry, no matter how bloated you are. This lack of nutrients will also mean you constantly feel tired, ill and lethargic.

You also have to get it clear in your mind that you cannot get round the problem with a multivitamin, or one of these synthetic 'meal replacement' bars that supposedly contain all the vitamins and minerals you need. How can something man made possibly contain all the vitamins and nutrients you need, when mankind doesn't even know what all the vitamins are? And this is aside from the fact the nutrients contained in these things are either very heavily processed or entirely synthetic, and therefore it is impossible to say whether they do you any good at all, let alone that they are as effective as those contained in the natural foods that we are designed to consume.

Do you know how much vitamin C dogs consume in their natural diet? None. Do you know how much they need? Exactly the same as humans. The fact is that dogs create their own vitamin C internally. If humans cut out vitamin C they will get scurvy and die, yet dogs simply create their own. The point is that you don't need to worry about what vitamins and minerals your body needs, and even if you if did you couldn't come to a definitive answer because many of them have not been discovered yet. All you can do is eat the foods you are designed to eat. If you do this, then even if an 'expert' identified something they say is missing, the chances are you don't need it, just like the dogs with their vitamin C.

For these reasons you cannot just eat what you like and take vitamin supplements. It seems irrational to me to spend years and millions of pounds researching exactly what nutrients, vitamins and minerals humans need and in exactly what quantities, then spend more time and money recreating these synthetically, then taking them in exactly the right quantities, instead of just eating the foods that contain these naturally. Either by creation or natural selection we have developed to thrive on certain naturally occurring foods, and the less we mess around with this the better.

Again, let's simplify things for illustrative purposes. Let's say you have a living creature that requires vitamins A, B, C, D, E and F to survive. It creates all these vitamins itself, internally. However, what this creature eats is high in vitamins A, B and C. Now we fast forward a few million years. It's not still going to be creating its own vitamins A, B and C, is it? Not if what it eats is rich in it. Equally, if you need these six vitamins only, but what you eat is also very rich in vitamin G, then over several million years as a species you will start to use, and even to rely on, this vitamin G. You have to get this clear. We have adapted to our natural diet. The only way you can be sure you are getting the right nutrients and the right fuel is to stick with this diet. As soon as your diet strays substantially from the natural diet for humans, you start to make problems for yourself.

## 10. Feeling Full

Interestingly, no one really knows what causes the physical feeling of hunger at a chemical level, what it is, how it is triggered or how it works. Fortunately, we do not have to understand it at a molecular level, we just need a good working knowledge of the basics so that we can understand.

Let's firstly divide our energy source into two: energy stored as fat and energy readily available (i.e. from our last meal). The body begins to store consumed calories as fat within four to eight hours from the beginning of the meal. As you consume food, the body automatically stores the first 1,000 calories within the liver and muscles for immediate energy reserves. This calorie storage is known as glycogen. Once the glycogen calories are used, the body then activates stored calories within fat cells.

So let us agree that the actual physical feeling of hunger dissipates when you have those 1,000 calories within the liver and muscles for immediate energy reserves. Clearly your body doesn't want to burn fat as these are the reserves in case food ever becomes scarce, and in any event I am sure everyone is well aware that it is possible to feel hunger even if you have ample fat stores that could be burned for energy.

As these 1,000 calories dissipate, a feeling of hunger will slowly build up. How quickly those calories are burned up will depend on the individual and what activities, if any, they are undertaking at the time. When the 1,000 calories of readily available energy are used up we will feel hungry, and our body will also then start using up fat stores.

However, it is not as simple as just feeling hungry or not hungry. There is also a feeling of 'fullness'. This is an actual physical feeling of having food inside you. It can take 30 hours for your body to fully digest food, from consuming it to excreting the waste product (some foods are processed far quicker and we will move on to this aspect in a later chapter), so it is possible to have whatever you eat in an entire day inside you at any one time. So three full meals along with accompanying snacks all inside you. In this case that feeling of 'fullness' will progress into a feeling of discomfort; after all, if you have too much food inside you, you will feel uncomfortably full.

So it is possible to have a physical feeling of fullness and a feeling of hunger at the same time. If you eat a big meal you can feel full for some time after this, long after the readily available calories have been used up, and at this stage you can feel both physically full and hungry at the same time.

This problem is exacerbated because if we feel something for an extended period of time it ceases to impact our conscious mind. Are you wearing clothes and/or shoes now? If you think about it you can physically feel them, particularly when you move, but how often are you consciously aware of the feel of clothes in an average day? I am not talking about how you feel wearing them and how you think you look and how it impacts your self-image, I am talking about the actual physical feel of the material against your skin. The feeling is there, but it just doesn't impact your conscious mind. Because it is constant it ceases to register.

If you are eating three meals a day of food that is difficult to digest, you will have a constant feeling of fullness that no longer impacts your conscious mind. You will become largely immune to it. However, it is still there and it will impact your quality of life. It will disturb your sleep, make you feel tired and lethargic, stop you wanting to exercise, and detract from

the pleasure when you do eat.

## 11. Just One...

I don't pick at food anymore. I work in an office and nine days out of ten someone will bring in sweets or cookies or biscuits. I never ever touch them. Because if I want one, and eat one, I will still want one. Eating something like that isn't going to make you feel full or satisfied; all you will do is give in to a craving, but it won't end the craving. The craving won't end until the source of it, all the biscuits or sweets or cookies, are gone. After all, it is not genuine hunger or a need for vitamins that makes you pick up and eat a triple chocolate cookie. It is the knowledge that they are there, preying on your mind. Like the old Alcoholics Anonymous adage that one is too many and a thousand is never enough. If something is sitting there, on a desk at work or a fridge or larder at home, or even just on a shelf in a shop, and you start to think about it and fantasise about it and obsess about it, it is purely the mental cycle of craving that is causing the desire, not a healthy hunger (and by that I mean a genuine desire to eat born of lack of energy and/or nutrients). The only way to end the craving is to finish them entirely or make yourself so sick from them that you physically cannot take another one (and how many that is will depend on what level of 'uncomfortably full' you are used to feeling). This is the very crux of overeating, with all its frustrations, guilt and discomfort. Theoretically you can just have one or two, but do you really think having one ends the craving, or are you just craving, giving in, craving again but then not giving in the second time? And if it doesn't end the craving, why have it? For the two or three seconds of 'pleasure' you get when you are actually eating it? But isn't this totally outbalanced by the feeling of guilt, discomfort and frustration that accompany all such eating?

In fact, having one actually makes it harder to resist the second. If there are cookies on the filing cabinet at the end of the line of desks and I fancy one, I'm fine to not have one because I know having one won't stop me wanting one and the downside far outweighs the 'pleasure', even on a very short-term basis. I am perfectly happy to sit there and not have one. But if I were to have one the craving would increase dramatically for three very good reasons. Firstly, if you give in you give in. If you can't resist one how on earth can you expect to resist the next, and the next, and the next? Secondly, the craving will dramatically increase once you've actually tasted the object of your desire – the actual taste of it will fuel the craving. As I have mentioned, a craving is essentially fantasising about something, it is about imagining it. Imagination relies partly on memory (we remember having or doing something in the past, so we imagine what it will be like to do it again). The fresher the memory, the more vividly we imagine it, the more torturous the craving. If you have literally just eaten something then the memory of the taste of it is as fresh as it can be, thus the craving is at its keenest. Finally, if what you are eating is sweet and laced with refined sugar then you get the refined sugar rush followed by the low blood sugar (as dealt with previously) which is going to make you want another one even more than before you ate one in the first place.

Again, this is a point that is worth fixing very firmly in your mind. Get it straight that having one won't stop you wanting one; if you have one, the most likely result is to keep having them until you feel sick, or stopping midway when you will want the next one even more than you wanted the last.

If you are genuinely hungry (i.e. you are getting low on calories and/or getting low on nutrients) then eating something healthy and nutritious will satisfy that hunger. You will feel hungry, the energy/nutrients will be topped up, and the hunger will dissipate. However, if the desire to eat is born only of a craving, then it exists because something has started to prey on your mind – it is taking up your thoughts and you are thinking about it and fantasising about it. Will eating it stop you thinking about it? Will eating it stop you fantasising about it? In fact, eating it is going to make you fantasise about it and think about it all the more.

This is a useful point to keep in the forefront of your mind when this sort of situation arises. Most people will eat in these situations on the basis that they will have 'just one', so it is useful to recognise and understand why it won't be 'just one'.

It can be even harder to resist when whatever is on offer will be thrown away if it isn't eaten, like a pack of donuts brought in to an office on a Friday that won't last until the following Monday. Then you are not just faced with 'Go on, have one', but 'Go on, have one, or they'll be thrown away'.

Most people have an inherent reluctance to waste anything, particularly food. This can often be the thing to turn a 'no' into a 'yes'. Let's now delve a bit deeper into this aspect.

## 12. Wasting Food

My parents grew up in London the aftermath of the Second World War, and they both still remember rationing. Because of the blockades of British ports during the war there was a shortage of food, so everything was rationed. Everyone was issued with a booklet and you were only allowed a certain amount of each type of food. There were understandably very strict rules in every household about not wasting food.

In fact, even without rationing most people don't like wasting anything, food included. Most people have to work hard for their money and avoid wasting it wherever possible. Even among affluent people there is a sensible reluctance to waste things; more and more these days we are becoming aware of the limited nature of the world's resources, and the problem with dealing with the huge amount of waste products being churned out by the human race. It is both sensible and responsible to make good use of everything we have.

think of throwing food away as a waste, and of course at a simple level it is. Sometimes we can store excess food until the following day or a subsequent meal, but sometimes this is impractical. It may be that we already have our meals planned for the following day, or it is not safe from a food hygiene perspective to save it, or it is simply not as appealing the following day. In this case the choice is simple: eat it or throw it.

We have this rather strange view that throwing food away is wasting it, and eating it is using it, and therefore not wasting it, but if you think about it this isn't really the case. Isn't eating something you don't want just as much of a waste as throwing it away? In fact, isn't eating it the worst option? Once there is left over food on your plate the 'waste' has already taken place. You can't put the vegetables back in the soil or give the meat back to the animal and bring it back to life; you can't give leftover food that is sitting on your plate to someone less fortunate than you. By eating it, all you are doing is taking on excess calories and gaining fat from it, putting additional pressure on your digestive system, increasing your lethargy and contributing to even more health problems caused by overeating. Isn't this worse than just throwing it away?

Imagine if you had an old armchair that you didn't want anymore, that was too battered to sell or even be used by anyone else. Would you consider eating it to save 'wasting' it? Of course not. Doing so would cause you huge health problems and would be far more damaging then just throwing it away.

You may think that this analogy doesn't work because eating food rather than throwing it away is the better option as it means you won't need to eat later. So let's say for the sake of argument you have 3,000 calories in a day: 1,000 for breakfast, 1,000 for lunch and 1,000 for dinner. You burn up exactly 1,000 calories between each meal such that you are using the exact number of calories you consume. One day you go out for lunch and have a meal of 2,000 calories. You eat half of it and are full after 1,000 calories, so you have the other half left. There is a general belief that if you then throw this other half away, you then have to find another 1,000 calories later on in the day, but if you eat all of it you won't have to find that 1,000 calories you would otherwise need for dinner. However, as we now know with our understanding of how our digestive system works, this isn't the case. If you eat 2,000 calories at lunch, your body will keep 1,000 for immediate use and store the other 1,000 calories as fat, which it doesn't want to use unless it absolutely has to. Between lunch and dinner you will use up your usual 1,000 calories and so still be hungry at dinner time. Obviously these figures are for illustrative purposes only, but the point is you cannot stave off hunger by overeating lots a few hours beforehand.

Eating food to avoid wasting it is exactly the same principle as eating an old armchair. Eating unwanted food is worse than just wasting it, as it turns waste into something that actually damages us.

I am all for cutting down on waste, and so far as I can I try to only order or cook what I think I will eat, but you are never going to get it exactly right. It would be ridiculous to make tiny portions and then just keep making more if you want it, so the only practical solution is to cook what you think you will eat.

Ever wondered why animals generally aren't overweight (unless they are supposed to have fat stores to keep them warm or they are our pets and adopt our rather dubious seating habits)? Or why some people are just slim, they don't follow any particular diet or exercise routine, they are just naturally slim? The answer for both is the same. It's not just that they are eating the right food, it is also that when they are hungry they eat, and as soon as they stop being hungry they stop eating. They stop whether there is food left or not. The key is that they stop when they are no longer hungry, not when either the food runs out or they are so full they literally cannot eat another thing.

The problem is feeling full is like any other physical thing in that if we experience it all the time or even just on a regular basis, its impact on our conscious mind diminishes. If you are constantly eating until you are really full then you get used to it, and you then have to eat slightly more each day to get that feeling of being really full. You will find that you can eat more and more and more. It will put increasing pressure on your digestive system and have an increasingly detrimental impact on your health and quality of life generally.

The good news is that it is very easy to reverse this process. You need to eat slowly, and consciously, and when you start to feel full stop eating.

Stop whether you have food on your plate or not. Just put your knife and fork down and walk away.

The following is an extract from the Finnish comedian Ismo Leikola's act, which sums it up fairly well:

'I think I have a kind of a strange relationship with food because when I was a kid my Mum always said that you have to eat everything from your plate, you have to eat all the food because there is starvation in Africa. And then I ate, every day. And then I grew a bit older and I started to think that, how have I helped the situation in Africa? I'm now a little bit overweight. I hope they are happy. I have done my best, eating so much. If I ever go to Africa and they look at my belly, I will say that "I did it for you"'.

In fact, if you think about it, isn't finishing the food on your plate worsening the situation? Eating food you don't need does you harm and gives you no benefit. It's not even like you will actually enjoy eating it: eating food when you are full is frustrating and unpleasant, even if it is a food that you would ordinarily enjoy. The natural tendency, and we see this in children, is to eat until you are no longer hungry, then just stop.

We have to learn to keep eating, to eat when we are not hungry and even to eat when we feel increasingly full. And we do learn this, we learn it all too well. We learn to eat until we are uncomfortably full instead of just no longer hungry, or even just slightly full. We learn to overeat, we learn to eat larger meals, we get fat, we cause ourselves health problems and, ultimately, does this overeating waste more or less food? Isn't training an entire population of people to eat everything that is put in front of them, to eat to excess, to eat even when they stop feeling hungry and to keep eating even when they are actively full, wasting far more food than if you were to have a population of people who eat until they are no longer hungry and then stop? If you are used to eating until you are so full you literally cannot eat any more, aren't you going to consume far, far more food in the course of your lifetime than if you relearn what you instinctively knew as a child: to stop eating when you are no longer hungry, or when you start to feel slightly full? If you eat until you are uncomfortably full then you will order more food at restaurants, prepare larger meals at home, generally you will eat far more food, than if you just stop when you are no longer hungry and save the leftovers for another meal, or even throw them in the bin.

For me this was one of the hardest steps of improving my eating habits: stopping eating when you are full rather than when the food has all gone. Fortunately, it is a step you can take in very small increments. Firstly, start eating a bit slower. When you eat it can take up to 20 minutes to actually feel the effects of the food (in other words to stop feeling hungry, and to start feeling full). This is because the food has to go inside you and to start to get digested so that you start to absorb the nutrients and the calories, as it is this that makes you feel full.

As we've touched on previously, if you feel something all the time it ceases to register on your conscious mind. This includes the feeling of discomfort from overeating. However, just as you can feel your clothes if you stop and think about them, so you can feel that feeling of fullness (or not being hungry) if you specifically think about it. The process gets easier and easier the more you stop eating as soon as you start feeling full because the less you overeat the more you notice it when you do.

Think of it as a scale from ten to minus ten, with minus ten being really hungry and plus ten being really full. If you are regularly eating up to nine then you only really notice when how full you are when you get to nine. If you spend a day or two stopping when you get to five (and to do this you will have to concentrate and really search for that feeling of fullness), then you will then start to notice when you get up to a fullness scale of five. Essentially, the less you overeat, the more you will notice when you are getting full.

In fact, one thing that is really interesting is how quickly you can rediscover your feeling of fullness. Try this. Work out what you usually eat in an evening, and halve it. Eat this half portion and no more for three nights. On night four, try to eat the original portion. Eat it slowly and deliberately. See how much of it you can actually eat before you start feeling full from it.

With changing eating habits, the first few steps are often the hardest – after that things take on momentum of their own and become easier. There is a saying that a journey of a hundred miles starts with a single step. If changing your eating habits is a journey of a hundred miles, then this is a journey consisting of a short walk to the nearest cab rank, where a comfortable taxi will take you the rest of the way!

## 13. Hydration, Dehydration and Hyponatraemia

Let's start this chapter getting the basics straight. Every human being needs water and salt. Starve a person of water and they will die. Starve them of salt and they will die. The human body is made up of around 60% water. It's neither an exact nor a constant amount – the actual percentage fluctuates. This is because as we function we lose water. When it is hot we sweat; this is our body moistening our skin with water so that as the water evaporates it takes heat with it so that we cool down.

However, even when we are not hot we are still using up water: every breath we exhale contains water droplets so that even the act of breathing slowly dissipates our water supply.

Because we are constantly using water, our bodies have a reserve supply of it. Our organs and blood require a certain level of water – if that was all we had then every time we breathed we would lose precious water and we would have to be constantly drinking to make up the deficit. In this way we have a buffer: our bodies store extra liquid so we can breathe and sweat without immediately encountering problems associated with dehydration.

Thus, hydration is when we consume water so that we have enough water to not only sustain life and health, but also to ensure that our water reserves are fully stocked.

So what is dehydration? Dehydration is essentially when we do not have enough water content. It may be that our reserve levels are getting low, or that they are entirely used up and our water levels are getting dangerously low.

Most people are familiar with hydration and dehydration, but they are less familiar with the term hyponatraemia. Hyponatraemia is essentially when your salt levels get too low. It can cause you all sorts of problems and in extreme cases can be fatal. There are various causes of hyponatraemia, but the main one among otherwise healthy human beings is drinking too much water or extensive sweating. Urine and sweat contain salt, so every time you urinate or sweat you lose salt. This is why eating too much salt makes you thirsty; it is your body's way of getting rid of the excess salt.

Hydration and hyponatraemia are fairly straightforward, but dehydration is widely misunderstood and it is worth clarifying exactly how it works.

As we have touched on, our water levels naturally decrease over time and need replacing. This is dehydration. When this happens, thirst is triggered. After all, just as the body will trigger hunger when you get low on readily available calories and nutrients, it will also trigger thirst when your water levels need topping up. For most people in the Western world there is no shortage of water and other drinks, so there is no real need for anyone to become severely dehydrated. However, we've all heard the statistics about the percentage of the population that is dehydrated, so why is this? The reason is that the most usual cause of dehydration in the Western world is chemical.

Two of the most common recreational drugs we take on a daily basis, caffeine and alcohol, dehydrate us. They do this by interfering with the body's internal water gauge.

The amount of reserve water that your body holds is not a constant. Your body will gauge how much it is likely to need over a period and will reserve water accordingly. So, for example, if it is hot it will need more water than if it is cold (for sweating). This is why if you suddenly go from a warm environment to a cold one, you may need to urinate. This is the body dropping some excess water that it determines it is unlikely to now need due to the drop in temperature.

What alcohol and caffeine do is to interfere with the body's internal gauge so that it perceives that it has more water than it needs, so that it starts to lose water. This is why a cup of tea or coffee can make us need to urinate out far more than the amount of liquid in the actual cup of tea or coffee itself, and why we can have a few alcoholic drinks without having to go to the toilet, but once the alcohol starts to take effect we find ourselves having to go with increasing regularity. That is, until the reserve is used up and we go back to just urinating out the amount of liquid we gain from the drink itself.

So what people often try to do is have a cup of tea or coffee, then some water afterwards. Or if they've been drinking alcohol they will have a glass of water before bed, or as soon as they get up in the morning. This may seem like a sensible solution, but in fact it does nothing to remedy the dehydration for one very simple reason: chemical-induced dehydration takes some time to wear off. If you drink a cup of coffee, one of the effects of the caffeine is to trick your body into thinking that it has more reserve water than it needs, so it jettisons some. If you drink some water straight after, what's changed? The effects of the caffeine haven't worn off, so your body is still working on the assumption that the reserve water it is carrying is enough. If you then drink water, your body will determine that this additional water is unwanted, so it will immediately jettison it. If you are dehydrated due to the effects of a drug, you cannot rehydrate yourself until that drug has worn off.

So how do you know when the chemical dehydration has worn off? Simple: you will feel thirsty again. Your body will trigger a feeling of thirst when it gauges that your water levels are low. You won't feel thirsty when you are chemically dehydrated because your body doesn't realise that your water levels are low. When the effect of the drug wears off, though, the body will determine the levels are low and thirst will be triggered.

What you need to bear in mind is that when you drink when you are not thirsty, not only do you not gain anything, but you cause yourself an additional problem in that you are constantly flushing salt out of your body.

The other issue, of course, is that the two recreational drugs that are most commonly imbibed, alcohol and caffeine, are also taken in liquid form. If your water levels are getting low, and your body triggers the thirst mechanism, then you take a drink and it is topped up. But if you are feeling sleepy or groggy and you have a cup of tea or coffee, you are imbibing a liquid to get the caffeine, not because you need the water content of the drink. Likewise with alcohol, if you have a few drinks of an evening, you are drinking for the alcohol and not from genuine thirst. So we tend to be drinking more liquid than we actually need anyway.

What you need to bear in mind is that with tea, coffee, alcoholic drinks, and even soft drinks and juices, water makes up the vast majority of the drink. This water will hydrate you. But if you are urinating out any of this liquid then you are also losing salt.

So what's the big deal with salt? Salt is one of those things where current thinking generally is that too much of it is bad for you. Exactly what constitutes 'too much' is up for debate, though. There is much evidence to suggest that salt is bad for you, but no direct evidence. By this I mean there are lots of studies that take a number of people and look at their salt intake and general health, and there is a clear link between high salt intake and health problems such as high blood pressure. So the conclusion is that too much salt gives you high blood pressure. But what is not known is whether it is the salt that is causing that problem, or some other cause. Could it be, for example, that people who drink lots of alcohol and caffeine tend to eat more salt because the liquid form in which they imbibe their drugs causes them to lose salt, which causes them to crave salt and consequently eat more of it, but that it is the alcohol and caffeine that are causing the high blood pressure instead of the salt? Rather than salt causing the problem, is the high salt intake, like the high blood pressure, in fact a symptom of consuming too much liquid?

Human knowledge isn't at the stage of being able to provide a definitive answer to this. Some 'experts' say we need to eat less salt, some say we need to eat more. Fortunately for the purposes of this book we don't need a definitive answer. All we need is to understand four things.

Firstly, little or no salt is bad for you. Secondly, too much salt is bad for you (even the most pro-salt 'expert' wouldn't advise you to eat nine tablespoons of salt every hour). Thirdly, when your salt levels start to get low you will have salt cravings. Fourthly, foods that are high in salt tend to be calorie-dense and difficult-to-digest foods like takeaways, cheese, crisps, bacon, etc. Much of the appeal of these foods is the salt content rather than anything else.

So we have this balancing act of water and salt, and we need the right amount but not too much. What's the answer? The answer is simply to listen to your body. If you are thirsty, drink. If you aren't, don't. You don't have to avoid salt, just be sensible about how much you consume. Any prescribed guide has to be wrong. Think about it: how can anyone say you should drink six to eight glasses of water a day or whatever, or that you should only have one teaspoon or whatever of salt a day? The reason you cannot say this is because what you need is not a constant. Here in London in winter I will literally go from day to day without sweating. In summer I can be sweating virtually all day long (losing not only water but also salt). How can it possibly be that I need the same amount of water and salt all year?

It is also the case that many people need to drink extra water because their diet is lacking in it. Processed foods have very little water content, but fruit and vegetables have a very high water content. Do these six to eight glasses of water that we are supposed to consume each day include water in food? If so, then those who eat less fruit and veg must need more. If not, then those that do eat more fruit and vegetables must need to drink less.

I am not saying you should stop drinking water or start eating lots of salt. What I am saying is that you should know the basics and form your own opinion, and stop accepting without question guides and platitudes that have little or no scientific grounding. In particular, drinking a prescribed amount of water doesn't make sense and drinking too much of it can cause other problems. Listen to your body. If you suddenly crave a takeaway, are you actually just craving the salt? If so, isn't it far better to have something healthy with some salt on it, rather than a takeaway which will have loads of other rubbish in it, very little (if any) nutritional content, cost far more money, have far more calories, and end up containing far more salt than the sprinkle or two you would add to your own food? There has been a recent flux of articles in the UK press about the salt content of certain takeaways and calls for them to contain compulsory salt warnings, as they contain far more than you would add to your own food.

Someone once even said to me that if you feel thirsty you have already left drinking too late, you are already dehydrated. I don't disagree that if you feel thirsty your reserve level of water must have dropped – of course it must, otherwise why would you feel thirsty? However, as for leaving it too late, do you really believe that human beings would have reached the current stage of existence if they had to become dangerously dehydrated before they felt thirsty? If this were the case, we would have died out millions of years ago.

## 14. What Food Should We be Eating?

So what food should we be eating? This is really the million-dollar question. I don't think it is exaggerating to say that you could probably find someone who would advocate just about any type or combination of food on the planet. For every scientific study showing you should eat this or you shouldn't eat that, there will be a corresponding study showing why that previous study is wrong. For every expert advocating one thing there will be another advocating another. So how do we make sense of it all?

To me it seems sensible to just apply a bit of common sense. A point to keep at the forefront of your mind is that the modern world in which we live, in which humans have learnt to process, synthesise and generally mess around with the food we eat, is recent. As I've mentioned previously, in evolutionary terms the modern world has scarcely been around for a millisecond. The earliest fossils of anatomically modern humans are from about 200,000 years ago. Modern processing of food started about 200 years ago, so it's only for about a thousandth of the time that humans have been around that we have had processed food, and don't forget humans were evolving for millions of years before they become 'anatomically modern humans'.

For me it is a logical conclusion to assume that humans either evolved (or were created, depending on your beliefs) to eat certain types of food. If we stray too far from this path we risk causing ourselves serious problems, not only with reduced life span and weight gain, but more importantly with the quality of the life we lead. Food is fuel. If you put the right fuel in your car it works well; if you mix that fuel with other liquids that your car is not designed to run on it will not only most likely break down far sooner, but it won't run as well while it is running. Exactly the same principle applies to human beings.

We don't really need to become embroiled in a complicated technical bun fight amongst so-called experts (many of whom are funded by entities and organisations with a direct interest in the results) to decide what is best for us to eat. We just need to apply a bit of common sense.

A good rule of thumb for this is, the more something has been interfered with, the less you should eat of it. The more food has to be processed before we can eat it, the more we should avoid it. Conversely, the food that moves most directly from nature to mouth, with the least synthetic interference, is the stuff to eat most of.

This is a good place to start and gives us a good overall picture of which foods should form the balance of our diet: fresh fruit, vegetables, nuts, beans, rice, seeds, oats and legumes.

We can actually draw some confidence that we are taking the right approach if we remember that a basic indicator for all species is taste: foods that are good for us taste good, and foods that are less good for us taste less good. As I mentioned previously, mankind has confused this system by adding refined sugar or salt to things, and indeed by creating entirely nutrition free (and even actively poisonous) chemicals which taste like things we naturally enjoy (there is now a whole world of artificial flavours out there). When you think about it, this is really quite appalling, but be that as it may, if we look at the things we find the most 'tasty' we still end up with fresh fruit, vegetables, nuts, beans, rice, seeds, oats and legumes.

Now you may be wondering what on earth I am talking about, how on earth can I say that fruit tastes nicer than pizza or a burger? Or that nuts

92

taste better than chocolate? Or that vegetables taste better than chicken? But stop for a moment and consider the actual taste of them.

What is the taste of chicken or turkey? Can you really even tell the difference? Is it really a great taste sensation? Pork, lamb, beef: is there really a massive explosion of taste in the same way as with an orange, and apple, a grapefruit or a lemon? What does bacon actually taste like other than salt? Do you think you like McDonalds? If so, do yourself a favour and go order your favourite burger with no sauce. Isn't much of the taste missing? And isn't the sauce primarily a simple mix of tomato and mustard seeds? Isn't it the case that the actual attraction in most, if not all, of the processed foods we think we like is in fact either the salt, the sugar, or fruit/vegetable flavours (like tomato sauce, mustard, apple sauce, mint sauce, or other herbs and spices that are in fact just vegetables)? What does bread and pasta actually taste like? When was the last time you even had bread or pasta on its own with nothing to flavour it? And isn't pasta sauce primarily flavoured with tomato? Aren't the only bread products we eat on their own things like croissants, which have added sugar, or pretzels, which have all kinds of weird and wonderful flavours but even at their very plainest are salted? When you have a Chinese, where is the actual flavour? Isn't it all from the salt, sugar and spices? When was the last time you really tasted the chicken in sweet and sour chicken? You need to differentiate between 'taste' and your instinctive inclination to favour the foods you have been eating up till now.

When you start to really concentrate on what you're eating, you'll find that much of the 'naughty' food you eat just isn't tasty. It either tastes of salt or sugar, or if there is some flavour, it's actually fruit, vegetables, herbs or spices that give it the flavour. Much of the actual attraction with unhealthy food, when you actually analyse it, is in the texture.

A lot of these foods tend to be doughy, chewy and oily when we eat them, or creamy. This is the real attraction of them, not the taste. The healthier options are very different, being crunchy, watery or somewhat chalky (like chick peas, nuts and lentils). The textures are very different. So why do we favour one set of textures so much over the other?

There are two reasons. Firstly, and most importantly, the creamy, doughy, chewy, oily foods are the ones our digestive systems find most difficult to digest. These are the ones that leave us feeling bloated and uncomfortable, as if we've just swallowed a bowling ball. This is also the feeling we have associated for many years with feeling 'full', so this is the feeling we aim for when we eat. Fruit and veg doesn't leave us feeling like this, so we start to associate these unhealthy foods with feeling full, and find that fruit and vegetables etc. simply don't 'satisfy' us. Again, the real change from switching from an unhealthy to a healthy diet is getting used to eating until you are no longer hungry, as opposed to eating until you are bloated.

Secondly, what you put in your mouth is very intimate (queue the Sid James laugh). But it is. One of the things that repulses people when they think of eating certain things, like that infamous witchetty grub, is the thought of it actually moving in your mouth. Even the mere thought of that brings out the shivers in people. The mouth is an entrance into your body, and the inside of it is something we are naturally very defensive of. We only like familiar things in there (again I remind you that I am talking about food), so trying new foods or getting used to foods we are not used to is as much about overcoming that natural reluctance as anything else.

Start to analyse these processed, unhealthy foods. Really concentrate on the taste, the texture, and how it makes you feel when you've eaten it. Really try to analyse the attraction and see if it isn't just a mixture of either salt or sugar, fruit or other naturally occurring flavourings, and an association between texture and the feeling of bloating that we have become used to seeking out when eating.

In fact, this analysis of what food we should be eating also ties in very nicely with some other indicators, and some scientific studies that are less controversial or less open to debate or criticism.

We also have to make sure we get enough nutrients. As we've already covered, if we start getting low on a particular nutrient then we will feel hungry even if we have an excess of calories. So what foods contain the most nutrients? Well, the answer is the same: fruit and vegetables.

Some people struggle with the concept of eating nuts when improving diet, because people mainly view nuts as being a 'bad' food in that they are high in fat and calories. The point to bear in mind that nuts taste good and are naturally occurring, so we can be confident we are supposed to eat them. In fact, the fats they contain are good fats and nutritional for us.

96

And if they are packed with calories, they will just satisfy our hunger all the quicker. So you'll eat less of them but only if you are eating to satisfy a hunger born of either lack of available energy or lack of nutrients. If you are eating to feel bloated then you are eating volume rather than quality and, pound for pound, they are high in calories and you will get fat. Don't forget if, as a species, we have been eating something for most of our evolutionary progress (and if something tastes good and is naturally occurring you can virtually guarantee we have been, and by 'taste' I mean genuinely tastes good rather than just being something we have grown accustomed to), then you can eat it sensibly (i.e. not to the point of bloating) without worrying.

Nuts and their nutritious fat content explain our obsession with fatty foods. We have an innate taste for nuts and the fats they contain. We are preprogrammed to some degree to seek out fatty food because, in nature, such foods would have meant nuts. However, this can cause problems in much the same way as taking the sugar from fruit and adding it to 'food' that would otherwise taste unpalatable. Fatty meat, butter, cream, cheese: all these things are high in fat, but fat that we would never encounter in nature. Although milk and meat occur in nature, the real question is whether it would be natural for humans to consume them. It would not be instinctive for a human to suck on the teat of a cow, or to kill an animal and start eating it. If a cat or dog sees a small animal running around its immediate instinct is to pounce on it, kill it and eat it. Humans simply do not have that instinctive desire. Have you ever walked into a barn that houses pigs, sheep and cows? It's a really overpowering smell, but it is not a smell that humans associate with food. If we were served food that smelt like that it would repulse us, however to a wolf or a tiger, that smells like food – it would drive them wild with hunger. Humans simply do not react in the same way. Yes, I am aware that humans have been cooking meat since a very early stage in their history, but don't forget that cooking is one stage away from 'naturally occurring'. In evolutionary terms we've been cooking and eating meat for a very small percentage of our existence. Yes, we may have been cooking and eating meat since we developed into what we now classify as a human being, but we were evolving well before this. There have been some recent findings to suggest that giant pandas are not suited to a diet of bamboo. They have eaten an almost exclusive bamboo diet for about 2 million years, but they evolved from bears that ate both plants and meat. Still, after 2 million years, they have not properly evolved into their exclusively bamboo diet. Evolution is an incredibly slow process.

But what about making sure we eat the food that is best for our digestive system? For this we need easily digestible food, with a high water and fibre content. Surprise surprise, this is fruit and vegetables as well.

Now is a good time to explain a bit more about fibre. Fibre is an indigestible part of fruit and vegetables, but it is indigestible in a good way instead of a bad way.

We've already covered how, when food moves through your digestive tract, it has a long distance to cover, 30 feet to be exact. From point of entry to point of exit it travels 30 feet. We've already considered how it is the muscles in our digestive tract that push food and liquid through us. Fibre actually gives your digestive tract something to grip on to, which hugely assists the process of working the food through you, meaning the process is far more effective and efficient.

Fibre is the key thing that aids digestion. It cannot be digested itself, it literally gives our digestive system something to grip on to, to force the food through our bodies.

The other good thing about fibre is, because it is indigestible itself, it contributes nothing in the way of calories. It actually increases food volume without increasing caloric content, and so increases the feeling of being full.

If you are eating a high fibre diet then you will find that what you eat one day will be evacuated the following day. This will also have an impact on how much your digestive system (i.e. stomach) bulges out.

Now, before you throw this book in the bin because it is yet another book telling you to cut back on meat, dairy and processed foods, let's consider in a bit more detail why people become so animated over the issue of meat / dairy / vegan / vegetarian diets.

Some issues in our lives we will happily chat to people about, and if they have different views to us we will happily hear them out and even consider changing our own views. Other issues, however, are far closer to our hearts, so if someone starts trotting out a viewpoint that contradicts our own we don't listen, we don't consider: our immediate reaction is to go on the attack.

In his book *Freedom from the Diet Trap*, Jason Vale makes an excellent point that people become very animated when confronted with a vegetarian or vegan diet about where they will get their protein, iron, calcium and vitamin B12. But when they are on a fast food diet they don't seem to worry about where they are getting their vitamin E, vitamin K, vitamin C, potassium or all the other nutrients that are only found in fruit, vegetables and nuts. They also don't seem concerned about the associated weight gain, lethargy and sleep disturbance.

The problem, and the reason changes to our diet cause such an extreme reaction, is that we rarely approach the topic logically, and in fact the decision is being made by our innate tendency to not want to change our diet. We eat what we eat, we're alive, so why change anything? That's how we work on an instinctive level because naturally we fear the new diet may poison us or be worse for us. It's an instinctive fear, like jumping out of a plane even though you are wearing a parachute. One of my most vivid memories of my entire life is my first parachute jump. It was from a skyvan (which is literally like an elongated Ford Transit van with wings) which the RAF used for parachute training, back in 2000, flying over the A40 up near Oxford. It was a scalding hot day and the whole back of the skyvan was open ready for the drop. It smelt of diesel and hot air and sweat. I remember the skyvan banking as it turned to line up for the drop, so the A40 and the rest of the world around it was all at an angle and I felt twice as heavy as I was as the momentum pushed me down. The actual chances of something going wrong were minimal, but the level of fear I felt was possibly one of the keenest. The reason the memory is so clear still so many years down the line is that adrenaline heightens perception. My point is that I have faced many more dangerous situations than that parachute jump over the years, but little, if anything, has impacted me in that same way. Why? Because instinct is hugely powerful, particularly when we are facing a survival issue. All humans have an innate fear of heights. Of course some people don't seem to have that fear, but they lose it by facing it, for example by jumping from a plane so many times that they prove to themselves on a conscious, subconscious and instinctive level that what they are doing is safe. Diet is another survival point, and is something therefore we can often find difficult to approach rationally. This is why often when discussions take place about the vegan or vegetarian diet, it is often less like a group of civilised people having a sensible two-way conversation, and more like a bunch of gorillas throwing excrement at one another. Our instinct is a powerful and important survival force. Sometimes you do need to override our instinctive fears, and changing your diet is one of those times.

The point is, is our fear of changing our diet due to a genuine concern over what vitamins we are getting? If so, why don't we apply the same concerns to our current diet, particularly if our current diet is obviously woefully short on the fruit and vegetables where the vast majority of the vitamins and minerals we actually need are found? Or it just an excuse born out of our instinctive fear of changing your diet?

We've all heard the fact that we have a tenth of the hydrochloride acid of carnivores; that our saliva is alkaline, whereas for carnivores it is acid; that we have long intestines, whereas carnivores have short. All of this suggests that humans are not designed to eat meat. On the other hand we have canine teeth which, it is argued, act as the sharp front teeth for tearing meat.

Whichever side of the fence you come down on, I don't think it a huge stretch of the imagination to suggest that, at the very least, meat should not be such a dominant part of our diet as it currently is.

Please also remember that this book is about diet, and right back at the start I clarified that when I used the word diet in this book I would be referring to the food we choose to eat long term on a day to day basis. Not the only food we ever eat. Diet is not like drug addiction, in that it is all or nothing. What forms the majority of your diet will determine your quality of life, fitness, health and body shape. Let me get this point absolutely clear: I eat burgers, kebabs, crisps, chocolate, processed food and dairy. But I don't eat much of them. Indeed, I find I eat less and less of them, not through restriction but through choice. The times I have them these days tend to be when nothing else is available (for example if you go out with friends for a meal and end up at a steak restaurant or a pizza place). Through concentrating on the actual taste of things and by concentrating on how different foods make you feel after you have eaten them, you will find your tastes change. As we've dealt with previously, 'taste' is not an unchangeable constant, we tend to simply chose food that we are used to.

Clearly, if someone has a healthy lifestyle and has a slice of pizza once a week it will have virtually no negative impact on them at all. Conversely, if they eat nothing but pizza with one piece of fruit per week, they will be overweight, weak and exhausted. May 'experts' come up with something in the region of 70/30 (70% 'healthy' and 30% 'unhealthy'). The problem I have with this is it doesn't address the real issue: stopping the desire for unhealthy food, which is really one of the purposes of this book.

One of the things people are often concerned about when adopting a more vegetarian/vegan diet is choice. They say that a vegetarian or vegan diet is restrictive. Again, I think this is one of the illogical fears born out of our instinctive reluctance to change our diet. I agree that if you go to a restaurant the vegetarian choices are usually limited, and the vegan choices are usually non-existent. But isn't this really that restaurants tend to offer mainly meat-based meals? Look at it logically: if you are eating meat you get chicken, beef, lamb and pork. I know you do get some other weird and wonderful meats, but no one really eats these regularly (and they tend to all taste much like the other meats), so from a practical point of view you get the four. Add dairy in and you get milk. No one really cooks with milk, but you can add in butter (which is just oil and salt) and cheese (which is salt and the slightly sicky flavour of off milk). There are maybe three or four other types of cheese that people tend to cook with, the flavours broadly similar, but let's agree they count for different options. So you have maybe four meat and four dairy. These are the meat and dairy choices.

On the non-meat and non-dairy side you have apples, pears, cinnamon, oranges, lemons, grapes, banana, grapefruits, peas, sweetcorn, anise, basil, capers, blackcurrants, cardamom, pepper, salt, chives, cloves, cumin, dill, elderflower, garlic, ginger, horseradish, mustard, liquorice, lime, nutmeg, oregano, paprika, spinach, parsley, peppermint, rosemary, saffron, sage, sesame seeds, lettuce, onions, spearmint, tarragon, thyme, turmeric, vanilla, wasabi, marjoram, watercress, wintergreen, bay leaf, avocado, apricots, chillies, parsnips, mangos, peanuts, lentils, oats, coriander, hazelnuts, cashew nuts, blueberries, cranberries, potatoes, chicory, broccoli, swede, courgettes, cucumbers, olives, tomatoes, chickpeas, runner beans, leeks, black beans, kidney beans, pinto beans, black-eyed peas, broad beans, sesame seeds, brazil nuts, poppy seeds, almonds. I'm getting a little bored of typing now and am probably not even a tenth of the way through. Anyway, I suspect I have made my point. Just because restaurants offer mainly meat and cheese options, and because our own kitchens at home tend to replicate this, doesn't mean these are the only options.

One of the things that concerned me for some time was vitamin b12. I could see the logic behind a vegan diet, but if there was a vitamin that was lacking that humans genuinely need to survive, then surely this is proof that the vegan diet is not a natural one for humans? In fact, vitamin b12 comes from the soil. The reason meat is rich in vitamin b12 is because when animals eat grass or other plants they don't wash them several times before eating them, they just chomp them up, usually with clods of earth still hanging off them. The lack of vitamin b12 in the vegan diet is not so much evidence that the diet isn't suitable for humans, but rather that we evolved eating fruit and vegetables in much the same way that animals do, i.e. with the dirt still on them.

Now I am not suggesting you start eating earth (although some cultures do exactly that, and there are experts who advocate it, which really does prove the point that you can find an expert or 'scientific' study to support virtually any position when it comes to diet). My point is purely that vitamin b12 isn't necessarily proof that the vegan diet is not a natural one for humans. The other nutrients that people usually start talking about with regards to the vegan diet are protein, iron and calcium, but in fact all of these are perfectly adequately represented in fruit, vegetables, nuts, beans, rice, seeds, oats and legumes. Protein is a big one for many people. Protein is made up of amino acids. Humans actually synthesise (i.e. make internally) most of the amino acids, the remainder (i.e. the ones that we cannot synthesise and that we therefore need to obtain through our diet) can all be found in naturally occurring foods.

However, I reiterate that you do not need to go vegan, or even vegetarian, if you do not want to. 'Diet' is about what forms the majority of our food, not all of it. There are often other issues at stake in a decision of this sort that are outside the scope of this book (such as the humanitarian side, the effect on the planet and local communities, etc.). The remit of this book is merely to point out the health and fitness aspect. The actual decision, as ever, lies entirely with you.

## 15. On Your Marks...

How quickly do you tend to eat? There is a very clear correlation that shows that people who eat quickly tend to be more overweight. That may seem to be stating the obvious; after all, those who enjoy food more are surely more likely to eat quickly and therefore be more inclined to be overweight.

We tend to take this concept for granted. After all, think of your favourite, unhealthy, processed food. Chocolate, pizza, burger, crisps, whatever. What would your answer be if I gave you whatever your favourite is, and, say, an apple, and asked you which one you are likely to eat quicker? The answer's obvious, right? You'd eat your favourite food faster. And if I then asked you why, the answer's equally as obvious. Because you prefer it, you're going to eat it quicker, you're more enthusiastic about it. We tend to take this for granted, but if you stop and think about it shouldn't it be the other way round?

If you were planning and looking forward to having sex with someone, would you deliberately look to get it over with as quickly as possible? I appreciate it might work out that way, but it wouldn't be deliberate! You might be very enthusiastic about what you were intending to do, and you might go about it energetically, but this would not mean trying to get it over with as soon as possible.

If there is pleasure in eating, wouldn't we want it to go on for as long as possible? Wouldn't this suggest we should slow down, and eat as slowly as we can, to savour every mouthful? If the food tastes good, wouldn't we want to keep it in our mouths for as long as possible? After all, you don't have taste buds in your neck or stomach; as soon as the food goes to the back of your throat and the swallowing motion starts, you can no longer taste it. I appreciate that there is pleasure in swallowing food, just as there is in tasting it (otherwise you could quite easily lose weight by chewing food, but then spitting it out rather than swallowing it), but this still doesn't explain why we would eat fast. After all, if a meal can be divided into, say, 30 mouthfuls, then we are getting 30 pleasures of swallowing regardless of whether we eat the entire meal in 2 minutes or 20. But if we eat it in 2 minutes then we only have 2 minutes of taste pleasure instead of 20.

It is also worth bearing in mind that the more we chew food, the more broken up it becomes and the more our saliva is mixed in with it. Saliva is an integral and important part of the digestive process – it greatly assists the body in digesting what we eat. Given all the above, why on earth would we end up eating so quickly?

Before we fully delve into the reasons for this, we need to understand a few other aspects of eating and digestion. Firstly, we need to appreciate the time lag between eating enough to make us feel full, and actually feeling full.

Don't forget, part of hunger is the genuine need for energy and/or nutrients. But it takes time for the food to be far enough along being digested for some of these nutrients and some of this energy to be absorbed and put to use, such that you start to feel satisfied from what you've eaten. So you don't feel satisfied as soon as the food goes down your neck – it takes a few minutes before it registers on your brain (the timings aren't clear but mostly it is estimated to be around 20 minutes). Think how much food you can eat in 20 minutes. If you are anything like me, it will be a fair amount. So the quicker you eat, the more likely you are to overeat.

Just to give an illustrative example, let's say you are genuinely hungry (i.e. you need energy and nutrients) and one portion will give you the exact amount of energy and nutrients you need. You eat this one portion, you eat it slowly, giving it a chance to register on your body that the energy and nutrients are being absorbed. You stop being hungry from this one portion and all is good.

However, let's say you are in exactly the same position (you need energy and nutrients and the one portion will provide you with exactly what you need). However, this time you bolt this one portion down as fast as you can. The second you finish it you are still just as hungry as when you started it, because your body hasn't yet had a chance to register that it now has the energy and nutrients it needs. You're still hungry, so you have another portion, and you bolt this one down too. You now have double the energy you actually need, so this second portion will just be stored as fat. If you've eaten this second portion quick enough then neither portion will yet have registered, so you will still be hungry, and you will start on the next portion. Obviously, how much you can overeat will depend on how fast you eat – the quicker you eat the more you will be able to get inside you before it registers on you how full you actually are.

The second aspect we need to appreciate to fully understand the speed-eating phenomenon is that food tastes best when we are hungry, and becomes less and less appealing the fuller we get. You may think you don't have an off switch with food, but trust me, you do. You may have become increasingly accustomed and able to ignore it, but it becomes increasingly stronger the fuller you get. You may be able to eat a whole pound of chocolate, but if you ate another and another and another, and kept eating until you were physically sick, and then kept on eating, trust me you would soon find the taste repulsive. Now I am not suggesting you do this to put yourself off chocolate, because the next day when you have recovered you may well want it again (aside from ending up in hospital), but my point is that if you are hungry you will enjoy food far more than if you are already stuffed with it.

So where do we get to if we take both these points together (the lapse in time between eating and feeling satisfied, and the fact we enjoy food far

114

more when we are hungry)? Well, the fact of the matter is that you were aware of both of these aspects previously anyway, either consciously or subconsciously (your subconscious will have noted that food is more enjoyable when you are hungry, and that you have a certain limited time period from when you start eating to when you feel full). Whether you were aware of these two points on a conscious or a subconscious level (or even somewhere midway between the two), the conclusion is the same: eat as quickly as you can so you can enjoy the most amount of food possible before you start to feel full.

This tendency becomes more pronounced if we are already embarked on a campaign to eat every morsel on our plates. If we are determined to do this, and we regularly have too much on our plates, then speed eating is the logical answer. If there is twice as much food as we actually need on our plate, and we eat it slowly, the first half will be enjoyable while the second half will be an unpleasant chore. However, if we eat it quickly, before we have had a chance to register how uncomfortably full it is making us, we can eat and enjoy the whole lot. This is one of the reasons we tend to lean towards speed eating: we are literally racing the clock to finish the food before how uncomfortably full we are actually registers.

There is also another part to this. Remember that we have already dealt with the fact that 'hunger', as in a desire to eat, isn't born of one single element. Eating is usually pleasurable, and it is normal to seek out pleasure, eating can give us a dopamine buzz and we may be seeking this, the sugar can also give us a high, we may have a lack of readily available energy, we may have a lack of nutrients, or we may simply fall into the craving cycle. Hunger is made up of several elements. Sometimes we encounter them singly, sometimes we encounter them in various combinations. As we've dealt with previously, it is possible to have a craving for food when we are not physically hungry, or even when we are actively full. When you are eating to relieve a craving, you are not really eating for the pleasure of eating, you are eating to get rid of the craving so you can get on with whatever it is you were doing before the craving took hold. Indeed, if you are physically full at the time, eating whatever it is you are craving can be physically unpleasant. Either way, there is no point hanging around: get it down your neck as soon as possible so you can then get on with your life. So speed eating can also be a sign that you are eating to relieve a purely mental craving, rather than to relieve a genuine hunger. Food you cram into your mouth as quickly as you can while leaning over the sink or leaning into the larder or fridge is all born out of eating to relieve a craving, not from a genuine hunger.

There is one final element to speed eating that is also worth covering. It can also be evidence that what you are eating isn't actually that pleasant. If you eat an apple or orange, for example, you can pretty much chew it quite comfortably until it has entirely disintegrated. However, if you eat, for example, a piece of bread it can become decidedly unpleasant if you keep it in your mouth for too long. Soaking wet bread isn't usually something we would consider as palatable. Other foods as well become less pleasant, or even actively offensive, if they are in our mouths too long. We've already dealt with how many foods we think we enjoy are simply flavoured with the healthy foods we tend to shy away from. These flavours often disappear within the first couple of chews, leaving behind something bland or unpleasant. So if you have a mouthful of pasta with a sauce made of tomato, herb and spice, the flavour from the sauce is all gone after a some pretty tasteless pasta. Or if you take a mouthful ...... disappears and you are left with wet bread and mangled meat. Or if you eat a slice of pizza, the tomato sauce and salt soon goes and you are left with (again) wet bread and stringy cheese. Because of this we develop a tendency to only chew these sorts of foods a couple of times before swallowing them.

Needless to say, if you are eating something that becomes unpalatable after you've chewed it a couple of times, you really shouldn't be eating it. Going forwards, you should be eating slowly and deliberately, and really identifying what foods you genuinely enjoy and what foods you have just become accustomed to eating.

A final point to make before closing this chapter is to reiterate a point made at the beginning of it: that chewing aids digestion. Your saliva contains enzymes that break down the food, making the whole digestive process easier. Failing to properly chew food puts additional pressure on your digestive system, makes food less digestible, and increases the feeling of bloating.

## 16.  Hunger – How Drugs Influence Appetite and Weight

Generally speaking, drugs can be divided into two categories: stimulants and depressants. Stimulants (like nicotine and caffeine) stimulate us and make us feel more awake. Depressants (like alcohol) depress or inhibit nerve activity and make us feel more relaxed and calm. They both have very different effects on us but they both have a tendency to cause us to increase body fat. Stimulants tend to decrease or inhibit appetite. If you think about it at a basic level this makes perfect sense. Naturally occurring stimulants like adrenaline kick in when we sense a threat (hence fear making our heart rate increase). The heart rate increases in anticipation of the response required to deal with the threat, which in nature would be to either fight or run away. At a time like this we are not going to want to eat. As I deal with in more detail in other chapters, although eating provides us with energy overall, digestion (the process by which the body changes food into energy and readily absorbable nutrition) takes a huge amount of effort by the body. This is why we want to sit down or even sleep after eating. However, sticking with stimulants for the time being, we don't want to feel tired or sleepy when there is a terrifying threat staring us in the face, which is why stimulants curb our hunger. This is also why many people vomit following a trauma: the fight-or-flight response has been engaged and the body is freeing up all available energy to run away or defend itself, and isn't going to waste energy digesting food.

So it may seem that this is an easy resolution to our problem. Why not just take stimulants to curb our appetite and lose weight? This in fact is what these miracle weight loss pills are – different types of stimulants designed to curb your appetite. However, they don't work for three reasons. Firstly, they erode our fitness; secondly, there is sleep; the other is something called 'homeostatis'. The first of these elements is dealt with in a later chapter, but for now let's consider the second of these three elements.

Sleep is something we need in order to live. There have been numerous studies showing that lack of sleep (or lack of good quality sleep) leads to depression, cancer, diabetes and a host of other unpleasant things. This is just sound common sense if you bear in mind that sleep is when your body repairs and rebuilds itself, and when your mind digests all the experiences, emotions and events that have happened to it. If your body isn't able to repair itself you will quickly deteriorate physically, and if your mind is unable to digest and assimilate what is going on in your life you will quickly find you are unable to cope with things. Sleep is essential; anything that interferes with our sleep is to be carefully avoided.

The problem is of course that stimulants either stop us sleeping or disturb the quality of our sleep. This latter point is a key one for those who have a cup of tea or coffee and/or a cigarette before bedtime and believe it doesn't affect your sleep. It may not stop you losing conscious thought for a few hours, but it will certainly spoil the quality of sleep, with the result that you will not wake up feeling rested, refreshed and ready to face the new day (which is how you should feel).

Again, this is just common sense. If you are facing a threat, the last thing you need is to feel sleepy! But if you take stimulants to curb your appetite, you are going to lose out on sleep. This on its own is too high a price to pay, but in any event it doesn't work long term. When we have not slept properly our body needs extra energy to make up for the lack of sleep, so we start to crave high fat, high sugar (in other words high calorie foods) to compensate. We also feel increasingly less able to exercise and the physical degradation builds up. As time goes on, the loss of appetite we get from the stimulant is more than balanced by our increasing desire to eat high calorie food and our inability to exercise.

So can't we just take the stimulants early in the day, cut them out a few hours before bedtime, and have the loss of appetite without the sleep deprivation? Unfortunately we can't do that either, because of the second aspect we need to consider: homeostasis.

The brain doesn't just create and release dopamine and adrenaline, there are a myriad of different drugs and hormones that it creates and excretes. It releases these at exactly the right time and in exactly the right quantities to maintain a delicate internal balance. This delicate balance is known as 'homeostasis'. The brain will seek to maintain homeostasis, so if you introduce an external drug the brain will seek to counter it. Therefore, if you introduce a stimulant, your brain will seek to counter it. It does this by withholding its own stimulants. If, for example, you just drink coffee in the morning, you will feel more awake and less hungry during the morning, but you will then feel correspondingly tired and hungry in the afternoon. You will not consume fewer calories, you'll just end up consuming them in a far shorter period much later in the day.

The other point of course is that the brain soon gets used to the regular morning hit of caffeine, so it starts to withhold its own stimulant that it would otherwise be releasing in the morning to wake you up. This is why caffeine drinkers need their morning hit to feel normal, whereas those who don't drink caffeine (like children) feel fine and awake and ready to go without it. This is true of every drug. The first few times we take it, it may make a difference, but we soon get used to it and need the hit just to feel normal. We have to take more and more if it to get the same effect. After a very short space of time, the stimulant ceases to curb your appetite anyway, or you end up taking larger and larger quantities to get the same effect.

With depressants, it's even easier to see how they increase our body fat. The most common depressant, alcohol, is not only an appetite stimulant, but it also contains a huge number of calories itself. It also usually leaves us feeling hungover and therefore unable to exercise. Alcohol not only stimulates appetite, it also anaesthetises the receptors that tell us we are feeling full, making us even more likely to overeat. Alcohol is also an energy source in its own right, but one that cannot be stored as fat. Again this may seem ideal, as we can drink as much as we like and never get fat, but unfortunately it is not as simple as this. Firstly, because the body cannot store the energy from alcohol it has to use it up, and it usually does this by turning it into heat (this is why we get warm when we drink). As the body is already dealing with an excess of energy, it is far more likely to store any other energy from any other source as fat. Also, alcoholic drinks are not just pure alcohol, they also contain large amounts of sugar, and this sugar is likely to be stored as fat. If we then factor in that we usually eat when we drink alcohol, and that alcohol makes us hungrier and less able to determine when we are full, you can see that drinking is a sure way to destroy a weight loss routine.

So even on a very basic level, taking drugs makes weight loss harder. However, they do something else as well that negatively affects an attempt to lose weight: they erode fitness.

## 17. Drugs and Fitness

Ever wondered what fitness actually is? What the physical difference is between someone who is 'fit' and someone who is 'unfit'? It's not muscle; look at long distance runners who are lean and slight but clearly hugely fit. Interestingly, the main element of 'fitness' is in the blood.

Blood is made up of red blood cells, which carry oxygen and other nutrients around the body to muscles and organs in order to sustain them. Every time your heart pumps, these blood cells are carried through the body to provide their life-giving nutrients to every part of the body.

When you exercise, your muscles need more oxygen to work, so your heart pumps faster to increase the blood supply, which means more blood cells can deliver their oxygen to your muscles. This is also why you breathe faster when you exercise – it is all about getting as much oxygen to your muscles as possible so they can keep working. If your body cannot get the oxygen around your body fast enough, you'll start to slow down and eventually you will faint as the oxygen level in your blood gets too low for the brain to function. It's a failsafe mechanism to stop you exercising at a level that is too high for your body to cope with.

In this, as in other areas, the body and brain adapt. If you exercise regularly in a way that increases your breathing and heart rate, the blood changes in two ways. Firstly, the red blood cells start to bunch up more, becoming closer together, so there are more of them in each fluid ounce of blood. Secondly, the age of the red blood cells decreases – they literally die off and are replaced much sooner, with the result that the average age of the red blood cells decreases. Why does this happen? Well, younger red blood cells are more efficient at carrying oxygen and nutrients – they can literally carry more of them.

The result of these two changes means that every fluid ounce of blood carries more nutrients and oxygen, so the heart doesn't have to work as hard to get the same amount of oxygen round the body. In this way you can exercise at higher and higher levels; in other words you become fitter.

The knock-on effect of this is that when you are not exercising your heart rate will slow down to lower and lower levels. As each pump of the heart delivers more nutrients and oxygen, your heart needs to pump less often when you are at rest. This is why resting heart rate (the number of times your heart beats in one minute when you are resting) is used to measure general health. The lower it is, the better shape you are in.

As you can see, the more you exercise, the fitter you get. It also of course works the other way: exercise less and your fitness will erode. If you sit there all day doing nothing your body doesn't need to use the nutrients and oxygen, so the red blood cells start to spread out and their average age increases. However, there is a far more effective way of eroding fitness. If you increase your heart rate artificially (i.e. without exercising) then your muscles and organs are being provided with an excess of oxygen and nutrients, so the red blood cells start to spread out and the average age of them increases at a far greater speed.

Why on earth would you want to do this? And even if you were mad enough to want to, how can you increase your heart rate without exercising? The answer to both these questions is the same: DRUGS. Both stimulants and depressants increase our heart rate without the associated physical activity, with the result that taking them actually erodes our fitness. So if we've already established that exercise just makes us hungrier, and isn't an answer to losing weight, why are we even worrying about it? Well, let's now turn our minds to body composition.

## 18. Body Composition

Most people, when they talk about losing weight, are really talking about changing their body shape. After all, if losing weight was the only goal they could just have a limb or two removed. What they are really talking about is losing body fat. Some people talk about 'toning up', but all this means is losing some fat and increasing muscle definition. To give an example, people often talk about getting a six pack. Everyone has a six pack. A six pack refers to six of the abdominal muscles covering the stomach area. Everyone has these muscles, it's just that for most people these muscles are not very developed and are usually covered in a layer of body fat so that they are not individually discernible.

Let's think about body composition. Starting from the inside and working out, you have your skeleton and organs, then muscles, then body fat, then skin on top. The body fat lies just beneath the skin and lies over the muscle. Therefore, if you want to look 'toned' (i.e. slim, with muscles that are clearly definable) then you need to increase muscle size and decrease body fat. Less body fat and more muscle gives you a toned look. Being fit and eating properly is the only way of achieving this.

Many people want to lose fat from a certain area, like their stomach or thighs. Your body stores fat just under the skin, but in certain areas more than others. In men the body stores fat predominantly on the stomach and round the sides of the torso (the love handles). In women the body stores the fat predominantly on the bum and thighs. It does store it all over, but they are the main places. Imagine pouring sand over the floor from a single point above. The pile of sand will be biggest directly under where you are pouring, but the more you pour the more it will spread out, although the further away you get from the centre point, the smaller the thickness of sand will be. That is how you will put on fat, with the main fat areas being the stomach and sides for men, and the thighs and bum for women.

You will also lose fat the same way: the last bit of fat a woman will lose is off her bum and thighs, and the last bit a man will lose will be off his stomach and sides. The key is, though, if you are burning off more calories than you are consuming then the fat will come off in that order;

130

exercise will increase the burning of calories, but it is impossible to burn off fat from a certain area before another. In the same way that you cannot eat certain types of food to put on weight in certain places, so you cannot burn fat off certain areas with certain exercises. I will deal with exercise in a later chapter, but for now you just need to understand that fat comes off as it goes on. If you have six inches of fat on your stomach and two inches on your arms, and if you lose 50% of your body fat, you will have three inches on your stomach and one inch on your arms. This would be the case whether you were doing lots of arm exercises or lots of stomach exercises.

The other reason why it is worth putting on at least some muscle (apart from the improved quality of life which I will expand on in a later chapter) is that muscle burns calories without doing anything. Each pound of muscle burns 30 to 50 calories per day just to sustain itself.

Going back to weight loss, you also need to bear in mind that muscle weighs more than fat by volume. One square inch of muscle will weigh more than one square inch of fat. The difference is not huge (a pound of muscle will take up about four fifths the space as a pound of fat), but you do need to be aware that if you do decide to combine improvements to your diet with an exercise routine, you will lose fat and gain muscle, so the weighing scales will not tell the whole story. There are many convoluted and complicated ways to record loss of fat without using the weighing scales, but in fact the simplest and most effective way is to take pictures. These are the best and easiest way of recording physical progress.

A final point we need to cover when talking about body composition is a distended stomach, or in colloquial terms a beer belly. This is essentially when a person's stomach sticks out. As with other aspects of this topic, many people are concerned about this (rightly or wrongly) from a purely cosmetic point of view; they are concerned about how they look with a stomach bulging out. But again, and with other areas where image is the main motivator, there is in fact a health issue very closely tied to it.

Many people think that a stomach sticking out is due to the layer of fat that lies over the stomach area. This will certainly add to the issue, but often it is not the main cause of it. Think again of what we covered at the start of this chapter. Directly under the skin lie the fat stores, and under them lie the organs of the body. You can actually see how much fat you

132

are carrying by pinching a fold of your flesh. The skin layer itself is extremely thin; its thickness varies depending on the area of the body, but even at its thickest (which is usually on the heels of the feet) it is usually only about a fifth of an inch thick. So, when you take a pinch of your flesh, what you are holding is almost entirely stored fat. Whilst this will account to some degree for the bulging stomach, for many people it doesn't account for all of it; it is what is underneath that is the real culprit.

As we've touched on previously, when you eat certain types of food your body finds them difficult to digest. It takes far longer for your body to process them and they stay inside you for so much longer. We've all heard the stories of people who have died and had however many pounds of red meat festering inside them. This isn't just an urban myth. I've no doubt that some of these tales must be exaggerated, but there are many very well documented cases of this. In any event, it's not that big a thing to imagine. If you eat something and your body cannot process it, it will stay inside you. Simple.

What the distended stomach is mainly comprised of for many people is the build-up of indigestible food which is literally stuck in their digestive system. Much of this is meat, the problem being not so much the meat itself, but the quantities people tend to eat, along with the lack of fibre which helps the digestive system process food that is more difficult to digest.

This is the real concern people need to have if their stomach is sticking out. Aesthetics is really neither here nor there – the real issue is that it is an actual physical symptom of a long-term diet consisting of food that your body is incapable of dealing with.

The other point we need to bear in mind is how we store meat, and our body temperature. We usually keep meat refrigerated otherwise it very quickly starts to go off. Our body temperature is usually in or around the region of 98.6°F. Would you eat meat that had been kept at this temperature for a year? What about a month? A week? Most of us wouldn't touch meat that had been at this temperature for even a day, yet this is exactly what we do when we eat too much meat and too little fresh fruit and vegetables. Of course the digestive system is such that the comparison isn't exactly the same; many of the bacteria that would thrive on meat if it were kept at this temperature for a year are kept in check (indeed there would be no meat left by the end of a year), but you do need to be aware that a stomach sticking out isn't always just because of fat. You can easily tell what your own body composition is on your stomach by simply pinching the skin/fat on your stomach and seeing to what extent any part that is bulging out is fat, and what is actually your insides bulging out; they are literally distended with indigestible food that your body cannot move.

The term 'beer belly' of course is ridiculous. If it was purely beer, then the stomach would be gone the following morning when all the beer has been urinated out.

This point can often cause people to panic a bit. It is one thing to know you are carrying around a bit of excess fat, which could cause health problems further down the line, but another to realise the actual physical burden poor diet can place on your digestive system, particularly if you then factor in the various cancers that are linked to poor diet. If this point has caused a bit of a shock for you then please don't panic unduly. The process can be reversed quite effectively by adopting a healthier, fibre-rich diet.

Now we've had a look at the basics of body composition, how do you decrease fat and/or increase muscle? As we touched on at the very beginning of this book, losing fat is all about eating fewer calories than we use, and to do this we can either change our diet, exercise, or both. Gaining muscle and getting fitter, however, are far more closely linked to exercise. We've already looked at what food we should be eating, so now let's turn to the topic of exercise.

## 19. Exercising

Exercising, like giving up or cutting down on our drugs, or adopting more healthy eating habits, is something people usually reluctantly consider because they want to look good or live longer. Exercise burns calories and speeds up your metabolism. However, people actually exercise regularly because it vastly improves their quality of life. Sure, people may take up exercise to lose weight or increase their health generally, but people sustain a long-term exercise regime for one reason and one reason only: they enjoy it. If you like the sugar rush / dopamine high from eating, let me assure you the high from exercise is a hundred times more effective.

People often find that they jump from one problem to the next in the hope that the next issue is less of a problem than the previous one. People will stop smoking as this seems to be the biggest and most immediate problem, but then their drinking increases. No problem, because drinking is generally perceived to be less of an issue than smoking. But then their drinking increases so they give up or cut down on drinking, but then their diet suffers. Again no problem; after all, you can justify a few takeaways and chocolate binges now you have stopped or cut down on your drinking. But in fact all of these things stem from the same thing: when we have a problem we look to take the edge off it. We do this by drinking, smoking or eating. All of these things make us feel marginally better in the (very) short term (i.e. for a few seconds) but have a huge negative impact on our lives thereafter.

However, the reason we keep on doing them is because life can be hard and sometimes we just want to take the edge off it. And frankly we don't care if it causes us x, y or z problems, we just want a few minutes' relief from all the problems caused by this life we've fallen into.

The beauty of exercise is that it gives us this boost without any down side. In the short term it gives you a huge dopamine high, it increases reaction times, improves memory and bolsters self-esteem. In the long term it leads to weight loss, increased muscles mass and significantly improved health.

However, the main reason people maintain long-term exercise routines is the hugely increased mental resilience, confidence and improved mood. I would genuinely continue exercising if it had absolutely no impact on my health, longevity or weight. It is about vastly improved quality of life.

I agree that everyone needs a boost now and then. But why not take one that has no downsides? One that doesn't take far more than it ever gives?

So if exercise is so great, why isn't everyone doing it? Well, one of the main reasons is that drinking, smoking, other drugs and poor diet leave us feeling tired and lethargic. They interfere with our sleep, they ruin our fitness, they make us feel heavy and tired and weary. People who drink and smoke a lot, or who have bad diets, simply cannot imagine jumping up and wanting to get out there and get some ground under their feet, just to want to run or walk or cycle or swim, to just be moving for the sheer pleasure of it. If you cut all that out and start eating healthily you will naturally start wanting to move some more, your energy levels will return and as you exercise a bit more you will start to sleep better at night, then you'll start waking up feeling more refreshed and more energetic, which will mean you are even more likely to want to exercise. It starts to take on a momentum of its own. The first few times you exercise you will need to put effort in, but very soon you will want to do it, so no effort will be involved. Soon your mind will start to associate exercise with the dopamine high and improved quality of life and you will want to do it and enjoy doing it. Just as you can learn to 'enjoy' drinking and smoking when your brain starts to associate the drink or the cigarette with the short-term effect of the drug (thus being fooled into thinking that it is receiving a benefit from it), so you will very quickly learn to enjoy exercise. The only difference is that exercise is genuinely good for you.

So what is the best exercise to do? There are so many different ways to get fit it is almost impossible to list them all: cross training, interval training, weight training, running, cycling, fartlek (yes, there is such a thing), etc. But which is the best one?

I spent several years of my life in the 4th (Reserve) Battalion of the Parachute Regiment. It is a tough regiment with an equally tough physical test that you have to pass if you want to qualify.

When I was in recruit training, someone once asked one of the PTIs (Physical Training Instructors) what the best training was to get your fitness up. His answer was, 'Put 70lb of kit in a rucksack, find the longest steepest hill you can, and sprint up and down it till you throw up'.

We were all expecting some highly detailed and technical guide to fitness based on the most up-to-date scientific studies (bearing in mind the Parachute Regiment has one of the highest and most brutal fitness requirements of any regiment in the world), and that was the answer.

Now I am not for a moment suggesting that anyone should go out and do this, but the point is that exercise is exercise. You don't need to get hung up and intimidated by these convoluted, confusing and often intimidating training routines. Anything that increases your heartrate and quickens your breath is good enough. For some that may be running, for others that may be a slow walk. It doesn't matter as long as you are pushing yourself even the tiniest bit. However, I think it is useful to go over the basics of exercise because, like dieting, this is one of those things that is so flooded with differing ideas, theories and methods that the basic irrefutable facts that we need in order to get a good grasp of the topic tend to get lost in the general melee.

The information and guidance I provide on exercise in the following two chapters is based in no small part on the principles that formed the basis for the exercise routines I experienced as a recruit and trained soldier in the Parachute Regiment. Whatever you think about the military, there is one thing I will say about the British Army: it gets things done. One of the things I struggled with most when moving back into civilian life after my service in Iraq was the attitude in the majority of the civilian population as compared to the military attitude. If you give someone something difficult or problematic to do in civilian life, most of the time they will come back to you and explain why they couldn't do it. It may be a perfectly sensible and rational explanation, but give a solider something difficult or problematic to do and nine times out of ten it will be done. They may have to smash down a wall, cross a river or wreck a vehicle to do it, but it will get done. They are not the subtlest methods, but they are straightforward, practical and robust. There was a phrase that was used a lot when I was serving: 'soldier proof'. It could refer to equipment, tactics or procedures, and it meant being simple, robust and above all effective. The following two chapters follow these simple but highly effective guidelines. Will they help the world's finest athletes to claw that extra 0.0001% out of their performance that will give them that hundredth of a second increase in speed to win them that gold medal? Of course not. But will they provide a simple, effective, straightforward and efficient method

142

for the vast majority of people to make some considerable and noticeable advances in their fitness and strength in as short a time as reasonably practicable, and then give them the motivation to then develop their routines in a way that both interests and suits them? I hope so. They certainly did for me.

Generally speaking, there are two types of exercise: aerobic and anaerobic. They are different in that the actual exercises themselves are very different, and they give very different results from a body composition, mood and effort perspective, so it is worth dealing with them separately. Let's look at aerobic exercise first.

## 20. Aerobic Exercise

Aerobic exercise, or cardio, is something that gets your heart rate and breathing up, but that you can keep up for an extended period. Examples would be running, swimming, cycling and walking. What aerobic exercise primarily does is improve your heart and respiration (or breathing), or what I think of as actual 'fitness' as opposed to increasing your muscle size. Of course, there is some overlap. If, for example, you start running, walking or cycling, you will see some increase in the muscles in your legs, but the primary result of aerobic exercise is to increase fitness rather than increase muscle.

Another very important (if not the most important) effect of aerobic exercise is that it is this sort of exercise that has the biggest impact on mood, because it not only releases endorphins, but because it gets fresh oxygen coursing through every part of your body.

So which type of aerobic exercise is best for you? This will very much depend on your personal circumstances and fitness level. In terms of what is the best exercise for increasing fitness, there are lots of different views on this. Personally I see running as the best exercise, but then this is

144

because this is very much the view of the British Army. However, I do genuinely think it is the best. I have cycled, swum, walked and hiked, and I found running the hardest and to me that means it gets you the fittest. It is certainly the exercise that burns up the most calories per minute of exercise by far. But let's keep in mind that ANYTHING that gets your heart rate up and increases your breathing is good. If you are unfit to begin with, you will want to start at least with walking or cycling. Walking is obviously the easiest; cycling is good if you can afford a bike and have quiet roads or trails near you (and of course somewhere you can store your bike). Swimming of course is very good, particularly if you have any joint problems, but of course this necessitates access to a pool or some kind of body of water. What is right will very much depend on you, and if you have any concerns you should speak to your doctor first.

Although running is the best aerobic exercise from a fitness point of view, it is the hardest, so in terms of starting out / enjoyment it may not be the best one. If you can afford a bike, cycling is an excellent way to start. Firstly it is far easier – a lot of cycling is pure momentum and you can go as slow and as easy as you like. But the beauty of it is you can cover quite a lot of distance. I love getting on my bike of an evening and just going out into the world and seeing what there is to see. You can go where you like and explore what you like.

The one thing I will say, though, is that whatever you do you should try to keep it up for at least 20 minutes. Although the experts are always changing their views, one thing that I was once told that was borne out by my own experience was if you are doing an activity and have to stop within 20 minutes, your body is not fit enough to maintain it. However, when you hit 20 minutes your heart and lungs are managing to keep up with supplying the oxygen and nutrients required for that level of activity. When I started running I could hardly run at all. I would just run as far as I could then when I couldn't run another step I would walk until I got my breath back, then I would run again. I found my period of running got incrementally longer and longer by only a few minutes or even seconds at a time. But when I hit the 20 minute mark, the time I could run for suddenly started to get longer and longer in leaps and bounds. So do anything, as long as you can do it for at least 20 minutes. Do it for longer if you like, but 20 minutes should be the minimum. The aim is to be out of breath and increase your heart rate for that period. If you have any concerns then, again, speak to your doctor, but if you are relatively young and otherwise healthy you can pretty much push yourself as hard as you like.

You may start because you feel like you ought to, but very soon you will be doing it because you love it and the improved quality of life really has to be experienced to be believed. But don't take my word for it, try it and see for yourself!

The other benefit of aerobic activity is that it enhances oxygen delivery throughout the body (which adds to the great feeling you get form aerobic exercise) and (from a more aesthetic point of view) results in fat stores being more readily available to be burned. It literally lets your body shed fat far more effectively.

If you do decide to try aerobic exercise, and you've not done it before (or not done it for some time), it is worth incorporating two or even three rest days per week. These are days when you don't exercise. It is also worth trying to do it as early in the day as you can. The endorphin / oxygen / naturally occurring stimulants you get from exercise will leave you feeling great and wide awake. If you do it right before bedtime you may find it harder to get to sleep. Secondly, it's a great feeling, so it's worth doing it early so you have the rest of the day to enjoy it.

## 21. Anaerobic Exercise

Anaerobic exercise is exercise that is higher intensity. It is harder, shorter, has far less benefit for your heart and respiratory system, and releases far less in the way of endorphins. The reason people do it is to build muscle. Muscle is used for pure strength, so this sort of exercise makes us stronger. Strength isn't the only benefit, though – muscle tends to protect joints as it supports skeletal movement. If you think of a knee joint moving, with little or no muscle all the pressure is on the joint, and it is very easy for the movement to go off course slightly which can cause joint problems. Muscle will hold the bones in place and make sure the movement runs on its correct course. One of the first things doctors say when you have joint problems is to build up surrounding muscle to take the pressure off the joint. Muscle is also good to burn off calories, as each pound of muscle burns 30 to 50 calories per day just to sustain itself. Thus, the more muscle mass your body contains, the more calories your body automatically burns. As we've touched on previously, this alone isn't enough to help you lose weight, but if you combine increased muscle with a change in your eating habits the results can be startling.

So anaerobic exercise does have its own benefits, but of course the reason most people want to build muscle is for vanity. Generally, people (both male and female) feel that they look better if they are slimmer, but also generally people don't want to look skeletal. What most people are aiming for is to slim down, but also to have some muscle so they look toned and fit. Let me be perfectly clear here: the purpose of this book is not to debate the rights and wrongs of this, it is purely to explain weight gain / weight loss and also exercise, and explain the benefits of a healthier life. For me the main benefit is a vastly improved quality of life, but there can be no doubt that for many people how they look is a huge motivating factor.

As we've touched on previously, looking fit and toned is about decreasing body fat and increasing muscle size, and anaerobic exercise is the way to increase muscle size.

The most obvious way to do this is to push weights in a gym, but you don't need a gym to build muscle. In my six years in the British Army I think I did a PT (physical training) session in an actual gym twice. Push ups, sit ups, pull ups, squats – all of these things can be done to build muscle and don't require the use of a gym. I am not, in this book, going to take you through every exercise you can do. If you join a gym, the gym staff will give you an induction and show you how you exercise different muscles, and if you don't join a gym you can, within a few minutes, use the internet to find how to 'build muscle at home' and discover no end of anaerobic exercises you can do at home. What I will do though is give some tips on how to get the best out of your workout.

Firstly, you need to be doing between 5 and 12 repetitions. Any more than this and the exercise moves out of the anaerobic into the aerobic (i.e. it ceases to be primarily muscle building). If you want the muscle building to be most effective, you should be going until you physically cannot repeat the exercise again. You build muscle by showing your body it is not strong enough as it is, so ideally your fifth repetition should be the last you can physically perform. To be clear, you do not need to push yourself to this level, this is only to build the most muscle in the minimum time. Even if you just do it until it feels a bit uncomfortable you will make progress, just a bit slower.

The movement should be slow and steady, both up and down. You should be in full control the whole time.

When you have done your 5 to 12 repetitions, rest for 20 seconds, then go again, then another 20 second rest, then a final set of repetitions. So three sets, with 20 seconds in between.

With anaerobic, muscle building exercise it is even more important you have a day's rest in between. Your muscles need this full day to recuperate and rebuild themselves to grow properly. Over-exercising can in fact be counterproductive. Some people do one set of muscles one day, then another the next; others do one day anaerobic exercise and the next day aerobic. Again, do what suits you best. As you become more comfortable with it you will find you settle naturally into a routine.

A general point on exercise is stretching after. Again, the point of this book is not to take you through stretching exercises – you can find these easily enough online. Stretching aids recovery so you should always stretch after exercise.

This draws the overview of exercise to a close. There are, however, a few points worth making before we leave it. In the same way we get used to a feeling of bloating and fullness, so the 'pain' of exercise has less effect on us the more we experience it, meaning either exercise becomes easier, or we can increase the level we exercise at, or most likely a combination of these two. Also, as your start to associate, in both a conscious and subconscious level, the 'pain' of exercise with the pleasure of the dopamine rush, so how you interpret this feeling of 'pain' will change. You will start to enjoy it, to relish it, even to seek it out. And before you say, 'what kind of weird masochist would do that?', haven't you been doing something similar but far more destructive by eating yourself uncomfortable for x number of years? Do you think it doesn't feel awful to have your insides so stuffed with rubbish that these same organs are literally bursting out of the cavity in which they were designed to fit?

## 22. A Day in the Life of... The Bad

So far we have taken a very objective approach to the subject of diet and exercise. We've looked at how our digestive systems work, what different components make up a desire for food, the actual immediate effects of poor diet (which, after all, are far more relevant than how poor diet may affect us in five, 10 or 20 years' time), what we ought to be eating, and exercise. However, it is not only essential that we understand all these things, but for this knowledge to really be of assistance to us we also need to do two more things. Firstly, we need to understand how they all fit together. Secondly, we need to apply this knowledge to our actual lives. I cannot apply them directly to your personal circumstances as I do not know them, but I can provide you with a generic example to give you a bit of assistance to do this for yourself. You need to use your imagination to see what your life will be like with poor diet and exercise, and with good diet and exercise. We will start with the life of poor diet and exercise.

Let's start by waking up on day one. You have a cup of coffee, perhaps also a cigarette, and breakfast. For the purposes of this imagined example, breakfast can be anything that is difficult to digest. It could perhaps be the great English breakfast (sausage, bacon, eggs, back pudding, toast and butter, fried bread, beans, tomatoes, hash browns, chips and mushrooms), but it could even be pancakes and syrup, toast and butter, cereal or croissants. I am not suggesting that all of these are equally bad, but none of them are the high water content, nutrient-rich and fibre-rich food which the human body is best designed to digest.

We've already touched on the effect of chemical stimulants in the chapter on drugs, so there is no need to repeat it here, but there is one other point on caffeine that is worth mentioning. Caffeine inhibits iron absorption. Bearing in mind one of the main knee jerk reactions against a vegan or vegetarian diet is, 'but where will I get my iron?', are you ever concerned about what your tea or coffee intake is doing to your iron levels? And of course if your iron is low you will end up suffering from an almost continuous hunger as your body cries out for this very important nutrient that it so badly needs. Even when you are so full you can hardly move, you will still have this hunger. As we've touched on previously, this is one of the main tortures of overeating: a hunger that you cannot satisfy (or, to be more accurate, that you could satisfy quite easily, but not with the foods you are currently conditioned to eat).

Anyway, turning back to our breakfast, as the food is difficult to digest your body must funnel a significant proportion of your internal resources into doing something with it. Your heart rate will increase, your energy levels will drop, and even though you've not long been awake you will want to sit and do nothing, if not go back to bed.

If the breakfast has included refined sugar then you will get the sugar rush, very shortly followed by the sugar low, so those who are more likely to have a sweet rather than a savoury breakfast will get a short-lived boost, but even then the boost is more than countered by the funnelling of blood to the digestive system, to say nothing of the period after the sugar 'high' has ended.

You will feel uncomfortably full from what you have eaten – even if the actual portion size isn't too big you will still be left feeling uncomfortable because of the difficulty your body has in dealing with this ingestible food.

Of course, there was no useful nutrition in any of these breakfasts. Even if the breakfast included the mushrooms and tomatoes in the English breakfast, your digestive system will be struggling to extract any nutrients from these from amongst the jumbled melee that you've presented it with.

So you've had breakfast. You will then plod on reluctantly and lethargically through the morning. For those who've had the sugary breakfast, the sugar high will shortly be replaced with the sugar low, so they will very soon start craving more refined sugar, but those who have had the savoury breakfast won't be much better off. They will still be lethargic and tired, caused by eating food that their digestive system can do little with. So whichever breakfast path you take you will still be tired, and so more inclined to reach for tea, coffee or a sugary snack for that much-needed boost.

Eventually you reach lunchtime. There was not much in the way of nutrients in your breakfast, nor in whatever you may have snacked on during the morning, and of course your body will have struggled to extract any readily available energy from what you've eaten, so even though you have an excess of calories within you, you are probably only too ready for lunch for three reasons. Firstly, your energy levels are depleted because your resources are diverted in large part towards digestion. Secondly, those same levels are further depleted because your body cannot easily extract the calories from what you have eaten, even though it is very high in calories. Thirdly, you've had no actual nutrients, and as we know a lack of nutrients will cause hunger.

This is why many people find they are hungrier if they eat breakfast than if they skip it. It is this that has, in part, led to this bizarre belief that breakfast can 'kickstart' your metabolism and therefore actually cause you to lose weight. This goes right back to my comments in the chapter 2: The Basics. How can consuming extra calories make you slimmer? Let me emphasise this, because it is a key point. The reason you will be hungrier mid-morning and at lunchtime if you have breakfast is because most people breakfast on the wrong kind of food. It may be calorie dense, but it is neither nutrient dense, nor are the calories easy for the body to digest. So you end up with lower energy levels, and greater need to eat, than had you had nothing. If you are someone who has found this, try breakfasting on fruit only and see if you still have the same level of hunger mid-morning and at lunchtime.

In fact you are most probably still actually bloated from breakfast when it comes to lunchtime, but the bloated feeling will have all but ceased to register on your conscious mind by now as you will have been feeling it for so long, and there will be a form of hunger as we've dealt with above. So even now you are moving into the realm of the main frustration of poor diet, which is feeling hungry and full at the same time.

So lunchtime comes and you again have something that your body struggles to deal with: burger and chips, a sandwich and crisps (which is essentially exactly the same meal except that the crisps will have a higher fat to potato ratio than the chips, and the sandwich may contain a meat that isn't beef), pizza, pasta, whatever. You are then in much the same position you were in after breakfast. If you had any refined sugar in that meal you may get the sugar boost followed by the sugar low; you will feel physically lethargic as your body diverts resources to dealing with the latest onslaught and struggles to get any readily available energy from what you've consumed; and again you will have that uncomfortable feeling that accompanies consumption of food that is difficult to digest. If you did have any salad or fruit or fresh food with it, again your body will struggle to extract that from all the other stuff that it's struggling with. You may in fact feel even more tired after lunch because your body is also still trying to deal with breakfast, so it now has twice as much to deal with.

And so you then plod through the afternoon much as you did the morning. The question you may now be wondering is, 'why do people do this?' The fact of the matter is that, in the same way that a feeling of being bloated eventually ceases to register on our subconscious, so does the feeling of lethargy and exhaustion. It starts to be a part of our life. It's only when someone specifically draws your attention to it that you start to notice it. People live their entire lives without fully appreciating the immediate impact poor diet has on their quality of life. Do you ever look at children charging around and wonder where they get their energy from? That was you once upon a time. Can you identify the day when you changed from energetic child to tired adult? Of course not, it is a gradual process, so gradual that we do not notice it. But that doesn't mean that it isn't there, slowly eroding our quality of life.

The afternoon passes in much the same way as the morning, and you may or may not be snacking on sweet stuff throughout to keep up your sugar levels, but eventually you arrive at the evening.

Many people, when evening comes, will drink alcohol. Indeed, many will drink it at lunchtime. People will all have their own individual drinking habits and this book is not intended to deal in detail with alcohol; however, there are several aspects of consuming alcohol that are directly related to diet and fitness. Firstly, alcohol is an appetite stimulant, so it actually creates a feeling of hunger. Secondly, as mentioned previously, it is an anaesthetic and a depressant, so it also depresses the senses that tell you when you are full or bloated, which means you end up eating more. Thirdly, like caffeine, it inhibits the absorption of certain key vitamins and nutrients which, long term, leads to constant hunger. Fourthly, alcohol has an impact on our quality of sleep, so we end up constantly tired (which also discourages exercise). Fifthly, as we have touched on in the chapter covering the effects of drugs, drinking erodes our fitness. And of course, last but not least, it contains a huge amount of empty calories and refined sugar. However, this is not a book about alcohol, and I have touched only briefly on it insofar as it impacts diet and fitness.

So your evening (or lunchtime, or even breakfast) drink will give you a boost as it anaesthetises some rather unpleasant feelings (like bloating and tiredness), but of course these are both things you wouldn't have in the first place if you had a sensible diet and fitness routine to begin with.

Then you eat again in the evening (maybe pasta, steak and chips, pie and mash, whatever). Again, you are both hungry and bloated before, and even more bloated and often just as hungry after, dinner. Your body puts still more energy into the impossible job of digesting the indigestible, again you feel tired (and if you have drunk of course this will exacerbate your exhaustion), so very soon you go to bed and fall asleep. However this is not where the story ends, because the most damaging aspects of poor diet actually take place while we sleep.

Firstly, you need to understand that just because you are asleep it doesn't mean that you are getting the good quality sleep that you need to wake up refreshed, well rested and bursting with energy (and yes, that is how you should feel, no matter what age you are). Humans go through two

162

alternating sleep patterns: deep sleep and **REM** (rapid eye movement) sleep. Human knowledge and understanding of sleep is in fact extremely limited, but all we need to know for the purpose of this book is that what you need is not just sleep, but quality sleep. Quality sleep is when your body repairs itself and your mind digests all the experiences you go through. If you regularly disturb your quality of sleep you will very quickly deteriorate, physically and mentally.

Firstly, the caffeine you have drunk will be impacting your sleep. As we have touched on previously, it is a stimulant, so it keeps you awake. It has a half-life of usually between five and six hours, which means the level of caffeine in your body halves every five to six hours. So if you have 100mg of caffeine in a cup of coffee at six in the morning, by midday you will still have 50mg of caffeine in your system, by six in the evening you have 25mg of caffeine in your system, at midnight you will still have 12.5mg, and so on. And this is only from one cup of coffee drunk at six in the morning! Can you see how those caffeinated drinks you have been having all day will impact your sleep, even if you have had them earlier in the day?

Secondly, any alcohol you have drunk will also disturb your sleep. The mechanics of this are covered in *Alcohol Explained*.

Thirdly, your digestive system can finally divert all available energy to digestion. The muscles in your digestive system continue to work, and there is a frenzy of activity while you sleep. You may not be aware of it, being asleep, but it will have a direct impact on you, and the flurry of activity going on under the surface will have a direct effect on your quality of sleep.

Finally, and perhaps most importantly from a weight loss perspective, because the majority of the digestion takes place while you are asleep, it is much more likely to be stored as fat. Don't forget that your body will keep around 1,000 calories readily available for use as energy, and then will store the rest as fat. If your body is digesting effectively during the day when you are active, the calories being absorbed will also be being used up. However, when you are asleep you are largely inactive (apart from your poor digestive system), so these calories are far more likely to be stored as fat.

This is how you can be eating far too much in the way of calories, and indeed be carrying far too much fat, and yet still be tired and lethargic. After all, this doesn't really make sense: the more energy in the form of calories you consume, the more energy you should have.

Returning to our 'day in the life of', you will wake up exhausted, lethargic and unrefreshed. So what do you do? You reach for the coffee, the cigarettes, the stimulants to get you going. You are also hungry, because although you are still bloated you have no available energy, and you are also lacking in vitamins and nutrients, which causes its own hunger. So today you are even more likely to reach for the drugs, to eat too much, and to be tired and lethargic. And so the days run on.

The other issue, of course, is that all of these problems are accumulative. One bad night's sleep won't cause a problem for an otherwise healthy human being. But night after night after night of disturbed sleep will have an increasingly detrimental effect. One day with no proper nutrients again won't have any noticeable effect on an otherwise healthy human being, but weeks and months of it will. The bloating will increase; we will develop a resistance to whatever drugs we are taking so will need increasingly large amounts of them; we will become increasingly unfit; we will become increasingly tired, frustrated and miserable. And so the cycle will run inexorably on.

So much for the bad, now let's think about how different things would be if we had a different diet, and a different exercise routine.

23. A Day in the Life of... The Good

Let's now have a look at what lie would be life with a better diet and fitness routine. You wake up and have perhaps some fresh fruit for breakfast. It is easily digestible, with some slow release energy, and lots of nutrients, so you feel satisfied without feeling bloated or tired. You then do 20 minutes of aerobic activity, maybe a brisk walk or a run. You may even do this before you eat, but either way the exercise gets the oxygen flowing through your body and causes adrenaline and other naturally occurring feel-good stimulants to be released, and this, coupled with the dopamine, has a hugely beneficial effect on your mood.

You go to work, where you don't have any particular food cravings during the day because you have some slow release energy to keep you going, and even if you do get a bit hungry it isn't the overpowering hunger you get from a lack of nutrients, a sugar crash, caffeine withdrawal or your body being desperate for readily available energy in any form to assist it with the hopeless task of digesting the indigestible.

Lunchtime comes. You are experiencing genuine hunger so you will enjoy what you are eating all the more. Maybe you have a smoothie: various fruits and vegetables, and even oats and seeds, all blended together. Maybe a salad with nuts or lentils, or even some fish or meat. Or some soup with some bread or crackers or nuts. Either way, the majority of it is nutrition-, fibre- and water-rich, so it is easily digestible and, again, has slow release energy. Even now, several hours later, you will still be on an 'exercise high' which will last the entire day.

After lunch, again you don't have any particular food cravings, or any crash due to sugar imbalances. You are still on the exercise high, but it is winding down a bit now. You head home, maybe you do a bit more exercise before dinner, maybe you do it after, maybe you don't bother. You have dinner, which could be anything: salad, some rice and vegetables, homemade rice and curry, lentil chilli – the list is endless. Again it is nutritious, and it has a high fibre and water content so it is nice and easy to digest.

By the time you go to bed a couple of hours later your digestive system has gone through the initial digestive processes nice and easily, and all that remains is some nice, easy processing that won't disturb your sleep, won't drain your energy, and won't generate huge amounts of heat that will cause you to wake up hot and sweaty in the middle of the night.

You sleep well, particularly because you exercised during the day, you've had no caffeine or alcohol to ruin your sleep and your digestive system isn't spending all night struggling under the pressure of a mass of hard-to-digest food. You wake up bright and early and well rested, and because of this you have extra energy and find exercising today even easier and more enjoyable than yesterday.

Sounds quite idyllic, doesn't it? Of course you'll have bad days, but you'll have more energy, be better rested and simply be far more capable of dealing with these bad days. In essence you'll be far more able to take the bad days in your stride and find them far more manageable. And don't forget we've only dealt in these chapters with the immediate effects on our lives; we haven't even dealt with the purely aesthetic points of slimming down, of developing some muscle, of the pleasure of buying a whole new wardrobe to go with your new shape, and the clearer skin.

So what's stopping you from moving from the one to the other?

## 24. How to Make the Change

As you can see, the differences between these two days are extraordinary. If you think I'm exaggerating I would say one thing to you: try it for yourself and see. Give it a month, compare the two and see then if you think these preceding two chapters are accurate or not.

But if the one is so good, and the other so bad, why do we put ourselves through the bad? Initially it is done through ignorance. We eat what is around, what other people eat, what we are given, what we are used to. Most of the time we don't really think much about it. Although all the things that we have covered in this book are going on, we are not consciously aware of them. All we are consciously aware of is that we get hungry, be it hunger due to lack of available energy, craving, lack of nutrients or whatever. We don't even distinguish between these different forms of hunger, we just feel 'hungry' so we eat, but through ignorance we choose precisely the wrong type of food to satisfy that hunger. But even when we become partially aware of the process (most people at least understand that fast food makes them fat, and fruit and vegetables make them slim), we still continue on this frustrating and unpleasant downward spiral because we don't fully appreciate the immediate detrimental effect it has on us, and we don't really know how to stop. We have an instinctive fear of changing our diet, but more importantly, when we get 'hungry' we start craving, and we only know how to give in to cravings (or to suffer them in abject misery), we don't know how to defeat them. The only way we know to end the misery of the craving is to give in to it. Even if we understand the whole process, we can still end up choosing the wrong food because it is decidedly unpleasant to be unable to enjoy your life because you are obsessing about something you want.

So a good place to start if we are looking to make the change is to deal with cravings.

The very first thing to do is identify what you are craving. This may seem an odd thing to say, but if you are craving something healthy then go for it! You may be wondering how on earth you could crave fruit, or a salad, or some rice and vegetables, but as your diet changes you will start enjoying your new choice of food, and when you get hungry you will start to crave it. This is really the point when you leave the whole issue of dieting and weight loss behind, when you actually want healthy food and choose it over other options through taste and not because you think you ought to have it. That time will come surprisingly quickly, the human body and mind is amazingly adaptable; if you think about it, it would have to be for us to have reached the level of evolution that we've got to. So first things first, if you crave something healthy, go with it!

But what if you are craving something unhealthy?

Just knowing and understanding the craving process often negates it entirely. Being able to understand it rationally is often enough to end it. Craving is a vicious circle that escalates because we can't think of anything else. When you understand it you are far more relaxed about it, you don't panic and you don't become obsessed in the same way.

The other thing that will help with a craving is to remind yourself why you are better off not having something, why the 'pleasure' is false and fleeting and there is an immediate and very real downside. If you are happy to go without something and know you are not going to have it, you won't sit there fantasising about it, and therefore you won't crave.

However, there are things you can do if you don't manage to nip the craving in the bud like this. The first thing to do is stop and take a breath (metaphorically if not actually). As we've dealt with, a craving is a mental spiral – it goes round and round, but by its very nature it creates, and is increased by, a feeling of panic. So the very first thing to do is pause.

If you do this you may already find that the craving is lessened, if not negated.

Secondly, you need to positively identify what is involved. Now you have stopped and taken a few moments out, examine what you are feeling and see what it is made up of. As we dealt with in the very first chapter, the problem with losing weight is hunger. However, as we've then dealt with in the preceding chapters, hunger is made up of many different elements. Sometimes it is just one of these elements, sometimes it is a combination. You've only treated it as 'hunger' before, because all you knew is that it made you want to eat. This is what usually happens when you try to diet: you are hit with this combination of feelings and causes that we bundle together and think of as one word: 'hunger'. All those things together can be very overpowering (hence most attempts at weight loss being unsuccessful). But if you can break them down into their constituent parts then you can deal with them one at a time.

So what is at play here? Usually the first thing to check is if there is any physical feeling. Is there an actual feeling of physical hunger? Even if there is, that is nothing to worry about. As we've touched on previously, if your diet is even remotely sensible you will not be lacking in nutrients, and as we've also touched on previously, the main problem most of us have in the Western world is that we consume too many calories, not too few of them.

Now I am not suggesting you should start starving yourself, but what I am saying is that, unless you have already gone several days without eating, any feeling of physical hunger that you are experiencing is likely to minor and easily manageable. Otherwise healthy human beings can go weeks without food with virtually no ill effects. Stop and think about this feeling of genuine hunger. Isn't it actually the case that the feeling of hunger is in fact a very minor thing, almost just a suggestion that you could eat something rather than a raging and overpowering desire? If you are in any doubt, think about eating some food that you actively dislike. In your current state, if this was the only food available, would you eat it or would you rather go without? If you would rather go without then, trust me, you cannot be that hungry, as if you were you would eat it.

If you are genuinely hungry then your decision is whether to eat something healthy or something unhealthy. Healthy food will relieve your hunger, leaving you feeling satisfied but not uncomfortable, give you a good night's sleep and leave you feeling energetic and happy. Unhealthy food will leave you feeling bloated, will spoil your sleep and probably make you feel guilty and miserable.

When you stop and actually identify what physical feelings are involved, you may actually find that far from feeling physically hungry, you are actually feeling physically full. In this case, if you do eat something you are going to cause yourself to feel extremely physically uncomfortable, feel lethargic and tired, spoil your night's sleep so you feel even more tired and lethargic the following day, and feel guilty and unhappy after you've eaten it. And these are just the immediate short-term effects, without even mentioning the long-term effects of increased obesity and cancer. And what do you get if you do indulge your craving? Well the 'pleasure' is going to be fleeting, momentary, gone within seconds. And in fact even those few seconds of pleasure are likely to be severely spoiled by the feeling of guilt and frustration that goes hand in hand with overeating. Are you genuinely going to enjoy what you want to eat? Or are you going to wolf it down then feel guilty and miserable for having it?

If you have taken time to stop and think, and have gone through the above thought processes, you will probably already have short-circuited the spiral of craving. Whether you identity an actual feeling of hunger or not, and whether you relieve it or not, you will have stopped the craving. Craving is an obsession – it is when you cannot think of anything else but the item in question, and simply by putting your mind to work on something else you will have ended the craving spiral.

Don't forget that a key part of craving is fantasising. When you are craving you are not thinking about the reality of eating x, y or z; what you are thinking is pure fantasy. You don't need to lie to yourself or try to convince yourself that you don't really want whatever it is you are craving, but you do need to think about the reality and not the fantasy. If you do crave something you think you probably ought not to have, and decide (for whatever reason) to give in to that craving, then test it out yourself. Think about, and concentrate on, every mouthful: the taste, the texture, how it makes you feel while you are eating it, and how you feel after you've finished it. Did it live up to your expectations? What it a wonderful taste sensation? Or did it just taste of sugar or salt (depending on whether you were craving something sweet or savoury)? Fix the whole experience firmly in your mind so that, if you come to crave for it again, you can decide whether you actually want it based on the reality and not the fantasy.

Don't forget there is a physical side to this craving. Just as we become used to the feeling of bloating caused by eating too much of the wrong sorts of food, so we start to think of an absence of it as being hunger. Although the feeling of bloating is unpleasant, when it starts to go it feels odd – something we are used to feeling is leaving us, and this is a time when we would usually eat, so we have a physical feeling, not of genuine hunger, but of being empty. You are not actually empty, you are simply not bloated; i.e. you feel as you ought to, but to begin with it feels odd because you are not used to it. You interpret it as hunger, but it isn't. The problem is that you get used to eating until you feel bloated, and then if you try to stop eating when you merely no longer feel actively hungry, you feel physically different. It can feel very odd when you first eat a meal that is made primarily of fruit or vegetables, particularly if you are genuinely hungry before you eat it. You will finish it, you will no longer be bloated, but you won't be hungry. This is one of the main physical feelings you will encounter when changing your diet. Fruit and vegetables will satisfy your hunger without leaving you feeling bloated, but because you are used to feeling bloated after you eat, you will feel there is something missing. It will feel even more odd because you won't actually feel hungry, your hunger will have dissipated. You will get used to this, and very quickly, but it may be disorientating the first few times when you finish a meal and stop eating without feeling bloated. If you've been eating until you are stuffed for years on end, getting up from the table not feeling ridiculously stuffed will feel most odd, as will walking over to the bin and deliberately throwing any leftovers away. In fact it will feel downright peculiar. You'll be walking away thinking, 'Is this really me? Can I actually be doing this?' It will feel like you've stopped eating halfway through a meal. Which is in essence exactly what you are doing, but halfway through a meal that is twice as big as it should be is exactly where you should be stopping!

All you can do to do to deal with this aspect is to firstly expect it, and secondly (and most importantly) to recognise it for what it is, and what it is not. It is NOT a feeling of genuine hunger; it IS a physical manifestation of how your body is physically improving, and just as the feeling of bloating soon ceased to register on your conscious mind, so this, far sweeter but still somewhat unusual, feeling of NOT being bloated will soon cease to consciously register.

In respect of changing what you eat, if you feel happy to do this all at once then good luck to you, go for it! However, if you are someone who really struggles with the concept of enjoying fresh fruit, vegetables, nuts, beans, rice, seeds, oats and legumes, and favouring them over your current, processed diet, then you can take things a bit more slowly.

I was at a children's party recently. There was (as well as food for the children) food for the adults. There were fruit skewers (skewers with different types of fresh fruit on them), pizza, sandwiches and crisps. I started off with the fruit. It was genuinely tasty and enjoyable. Then I had

180

the pizza. It was pepperoni. When I concentrated on the flavour it really only tasted of salt. Same with the crisps. The sandwich I had was chicken and bacon. The chicken tasted of nothing; the bacon tasted of salt. The bread tasted of not much. After all, if you think about it, what does bread actually taste like? In terms of pure flavour the fruit was head and shoulders above the rest.

If you have concerns about making the switch then, to begin with, start really concentrating on your food. Really think about the taste, the texture, how it makes you feel when you eat it, how you feel shortly after eating it. Remember when we talked about the feeling of clothes? Don't ignore the physical effect these things have on you. If you eat something like a bacon sandwich, a cookie, a biscuit, a burger, etc. don't just then move on to the next thing without paying attention to what it has done to you (which is very easy to do in this hectic life we have created for ourselves in the Western world). Stop and see how it actually makes you feel, physically. Does it remove the feeling of hunger and leave you feeling satisfied, content and with no corresponding unpleasant physical feeling? Or does it leave you feeling uncomfortable, as if you've just swallowed a bowling ball? If it leaves you feeling uncomfortable then understand what your body is telling you. It is your digestive system telling you that this particular food is a struggle for it. My books are not about me telling you what to do, and they are not about me quoting scientific studies that you have to take for granted (and that may or may not be reliable in the first place – every so-called 'scientific' study is open to criticism and undermining). They are about encouraging you to think about things, to question things, to apply common sense, but above all to apply your own experiences. Do you really need a study of a thousand people to tell you that a certain type of food is hard to digest when you can eat it yourself and see how your own body reacts to it? Sure I have explained how digestion works and why eating too much of the wrong stuff makes you tired, but you didn't even really need that. You know from your own experience that eating certain amounts of certain foods makes you sleepy. What my books are about is questioning the views we as a society hold about something to see if they make sense, and if they don't then coming up with a picture that does. Really start concentrating on the whole experience. Get a couple of pieces of fruit and try them, and just compare the difference. Experiment with lots of different types of fruit, vegetables, nuts, beans, seeds and legumes. All the time, keep really concentrating on the whole experience. Think about all the things we've covered in this book. Persevere and see if you don't find that your commitment to unhealthy food is actually not so concrete as you originally thought. If you need support (or even if you just want to link up with likeminded individuals), I have set up a Facebook group: Diet and Fitness Explained.

The main differences between the healthy and the unhealthy diet are that the unhealthy diet will make you feel 'full' (i.e. bloated) in a way the healthy diet won't, and, to start with at least, you will need to make an active decision to beat cravings instead of giving in to them. In fact, these two points are really the two main barriers between a life of poor diet and fitness, with all its guilt and disappointment and frustration and health problems, and a life of good diet, with its energy, self-confidence and joy. And these are the only two things that ever keep us on poor quality food: the desire for that feeling of 'fullness' (which is really bloating, but we have come to associate it with the feeling we have to end up with when we eat), and the ending of the craving (which, as we have dealt with previously, only goes when we have eaten so much it becomes increasingly uncomfortable to eat more, as it is born of a vicious mental cycle and not genuine 'hunger', i.e. a need for energy or nutrients) which can be far more effectively ended in other ways. And remember, giving in to cravings makes them stronger; beating them makes them weaker.

Another thing that may also feel odd to begin with is going to bed. Many people find they eat fairly healthily during the day. They are busy at work or whatever and so don't crave food (their mind is occupied with other things, so they can't dedicate their conscious thought to craving). I am sure everyone has done this on occasion: you have felt hungry and then got caught up in something, and suddenly you realise an hour or two have gone by and you still haven't eaten anything. How long would you have lasted not eating had you not got caught up in whatever it was that stole your attention? Or spent most days at work eating loads, then having a really busy day and realising you've hardly eaten all day. Really this shows that a huge amount of our eating isn't due to genuine hunger at all, but just boredom leading us to thinking about eating which in turn leads to craving. Also, a lot of people find they are less hungry during the day because they drink tea and coffee, and as we've dealt with previously, when you take stimulants they lessen your hunger while you are taking them, at the expense of feeling even more hungry when you stop. If you drink caffeine during the day and not in the evening, you will feel hungrier in the evening. This is why there is a tendency among many people to eat fairly sensibly during the day, then to end up eating loads of anything they can lay their hands on in the evening.

However, even if you don't do this, it is still common to have a large evening meal. Either way, eating lots will make you feel sleepy and often we eat lots then collapse into bed and fall asleep. Even if you don't eat lots in the evening, if you've been eating too much of the wrong food for any length of time, by the time you go to bed you will be absolutely drained and exhausted anyway. It can be a change going to bed not feeling extremely full. Because you aren't overloading your digestive system with indigestible rubbish, you may well find you feel more alert and less sleepy when you go to bed. Again, you will soon get used to it. You will also find you sleep less. Maybe you won't be so tired at bed time, or you wake up earlier. This is a sign that your body is no longer struggling with digestion, and is one of the most immediate and noticeable effects of swapping to a healthy diet. You will literally start to bounce back this quickly. You may find, initially, that you wake up in the night or wake up earlier than usual. Again, this is all evidence that the huge burden you have been putting on your digestive system is finally being relieved. It will take some time to acclimatise and you may need to change your sleeping patterns. Strangely enough, you can spoil your sleeping pattern by going to bed too early. Let's say your diet is abysmal and you need nine hours' sleep at night. You go to bed at 11 and get up at 8. When you change your diet you now only need seven hours. If you go to bed and get up at the same time you will be in bed for longer than you need to sleep, and what you will often find is that you will wake up in the night for a couple of hours. You will need to experiment and see what works for you, but if you are still waking up in the night, and you are not drinking alcohol or too much caffeine, it will be worth making adjustments to your sleeping routine. Humans get the best sleep when they go to bed and get up at the same time, so you should, as far as possible, keep to a set pattern.

Again, as we've covered previously, exercise will also help your sleep routine. And if you are used to lots of caffeine and are cutting back on this, particularly later in the day, this will also greatly assist you in sleeping.

Another sleeping tip that is worth bearing in mind is that I have found it best not to eat too much fruit and veg before bed; the high water content means you will likely wake up in the night to go to toilet. Equally, you don't want to eat too much heavy food before bed because it will disturb your sleep. Try to avoid eating anything for at least a couple of hours before bedtime – bedtime is the time, more than any other, that you need to ensure that you eat only enough to stop your hunger, rather than overeating, and even at the expense of being slightly hungry when going to bed.

The beauty of improving your diet and fitness routine is that it is not about absolutes. It is about balance. It is about finding the balance that is right for you. Unlike drug addiction, which is all or nothing, diet and fitness does not need to be so black and white. One of the knacks of improving your diet and fitness routine is to accept incremental changes. Many people tend to think in terms of absolutes. They are vegan or vegetarian or on a diet or whatever. However, this can have a detrimental effect. It can make you be too hard on yourself. 'I will never eat processed food again'. Of course you will, but because you are thinking in absolute terms you then, as soon as you do have a bag of crisps or a pizza or a burger, give the whole thing up and go on an eating binge. We have already dealt with why certain reasons for eating are false, and giving in to the object of your craving actually makes resisting the next one even harder. But never compound the problem by giving up. Do you think your body would find it harder to deal with a whole pizza, or half a pizza? Do you think that one chocolate bar will do you less harm than four? If you do have something you think you maybe ought not to have had, then don't worry about it. Think of the calories you haven't eaten rather than the calories you have. By this, I mean the sooner you stop the better. If you have something you think you ought not to have had, you haven't suffered a defeat by that, you have won a victory by stopping there and not compounding the problem by having more. But one thing I will say is to concentrate on every aspect of what you eat. Let's say you're at a party and pizzas get delivered. You are hungry, you really want to eat, and suddenly you want some pizza. If you have it, concentrate on every aspect of it.

188

What does it actually taste like? Is the flavour really that amazing? Or is it just the salt that is the main attraction? Is the texture that great? What is it anyway, isn't it just chewy bread and oil? Does it satisfy the desire for pizza, or do you want the second slice just as much as you wanted the first slice? Does it leave you feeling content and satisfied, or do you jump straight from feeling hungry to feeling bloated? Has your heart rate accelerated since eating it? Are you happy now or are you just craving something sweet to give your body a sugar rush so it has some energy to try to digest the indigestible? You may well find your mood improves, but bear in mind that's the dopamine high you get from eating – you could have got exactly the same from something healthy and nutritious. You may well eventually end up ending the craving process, but you could have quite easily ended that anyway by going through the processes we've gone through at the start of this chapter.

If you do this (eat something you think you ought not to have had, but really concentrate on the whole experience during and after you eat it), then you are in a win/win situation. There are only two outcomes. The first is that, overall, you conclude that you would probably have been better off not having whatever it was you had. In which case, great. You have proved something very important to yourself, something you will remember next time you are in the same or a similar situation.

The only other outcome is that in fact, overall, it was worth doing. In which case again great, you did something that was worthwhile, that you were justified in doing and that you enjoyed.

Either way, once it is done it is done. Leave it. The worst thing you can do is eat something then waste time wishing you hadn't. Don't feel guilty and miserable. Remember, guilt and misery are two emotions that your subconscious can use to trigger you to reach for something to eat, and you can think to yourself, 'I've given in now, I may as well just completely surrender'. I say again, don't think in terms of the calories you've eaten, think in terms of the calories you haven't eaten, the ones you can still not eat.

Start actually listening to the messages your body sends to you. Your body speaks with quite a loud voice, but we've just become conditioned to ignore it.

If you are really struggling, go and do some exercise. Go for a run or a walk or a cycle. See if you don't feel better after.

## 25. Conclusion

As teenagers, many of us start drinking and smoking. At that age the most immediate thing to rectify is the smoking. Those who manage to stop smoking then find their drinking increases to unmanageable levels, so they stop drinking. However, then their eating gets out of hand so they look to sort that out. Not everyone follows this pattern – some never smoke, or find their eating is more of an issue than their drinking. In fact, there is a whole host of different ways things can progress. Partly this is because every human being has 'ambition'. When I use the word 'ambition' I am not using it in the sense of career, meaning wanting to take the next step in whatever career we are following. I am using the word in a far broader sense, meaning a simple driving force within all living creatures to make improvements to their lives. Solving one problem quite often leads us to turn our mind to the next. There is nothing wrong with this; it is both sensible and perfectly normal to want to improve our lives.

However, there is another reason we tend to jump from one thing to another. Whether you like it or not, life has ups and downs. We have good times and bad. Sometimes the bad is merely an irritant, but other times the bad can be very bad: it can be overwhelming. Everyone has these times. Some have more of them than others depending on their personal circumstances, but everyone has them. When we have them we quite understandably seek relief from them. We begin to realise that each crutch we rely on takes far more then it gives, so we give it up, but this just leads us to then relying on the next crutch when times become bad. There is a drive these days to rejoice when giving up a drug (whatever that drug may be: smoking, alcohol, overeating, whatever). We are encouraged to rejoice when giving something up, not to feel miserable, and, above all, not to replace it with anything else. This is fine as far as it goes, but in fact if you want to give something up entirely, and not simply give up one destructive crutch to replace it with another, you do need to replace it with something, in that you need to recognise that you have been using your crutch for however many years to deal with the bad times. You have been using it to give you that little boost to help you keep putting one foot in front of the other when things get really bad. You will need something when things get bad. It is all very well saying if you can change something then change it, if you can't then stop worrying about it. Life isn't that simple – sometimes things go wrong, we cannot change them, and neither can we simply not worry about them.

Everyone needs a boost now and then. The trouble is that cigarettes, alcohol and poor quality food all take far more than they give, and we feel far worse overall for taking them. You will need a boost. As I say, everyone does. So make exercise your boost. If you haven't exercised for some time then you have to try aerobic exercise to truly understand what a boost it gives. And the beauty is there is no downside. The only side effects are increased health, loss of weight, far greater self-confidence, hugely improved mental resilience and a happier life. I am not saying you will be happy all the time, no one is, but by making exercise your crutch you are using something that gives without taking.

To be clear, I am not saying you should (as people tend to do with drugs and overeating) simply hide from problems and not address them. You do need to develop the mental resilience to deal with life, but when the bad times come you need to know in advance how you will cope with them without reaching for the sugar, crisp, burgers, pizzas, chocolate, wine, etc. This is what a sensible exercise routine can do for you.

Someone once sent me an email to say they had given up drinking, they were really getting into exercise, but they were worried they were replacing one addiction with another. My answer? So what if you are, go for it!

In fact, exercise isn't an addiction – a healthy diet and some exercise is how human beings were designed to live. We are not plants, we have the ability to move, to walk, to run, to climb, to swim. Exercise isn't unnatural, it is natural. Doing exercise and using it as a coping mechanism when times are bad isn't addiction to exercise, it is living life as we are supposed to. We were not designed to sit, all day every day, doing nothing physical. The only reason people find the thought of exercising repugnant is because they have been poisoning themselves for so long they are in a constant form of illness. It is natural, when you are ill, to shy away from exercise. This is the body's way of protecting you and giving you the best chance of getting on top of whatever illness you have. Your body tells you to rest and take it easy. When a human being (or any animal for that matter) is unwell or physically below par in some way, they become timid and want to hide away. When they are physically well they become confident, adventurous and resilient. Again, this is just nature's way. If an animal is injured or sick it shouldn't be out hunting, foraging, seeking a mate or looking for new territory. It needs to hide away somewhere safe until it recovers its health. Conversely, if it is well and in top physical condition, for its own good and the good of its species, it needs to get out there and mate and hunt and explore. In this way our physical condition is very strongly linked to our mental resilience.

There's a quaint 1970s'/1980s' view that giving up smoking and drinking and eating fast food and then taking up exercising is all about vanity and trying to live as long as possible. You give up the 'fun' things in life so as to look a bit better and live a bit longer. This is absolute rubbish. It is about enjoying life, about living it to the full.

We've already touched on how taking a drug can give you a momentary boost, but as you get used to that drug you need it just to feel normal. This, along with the physical degradation that accompanies any long-term drug addiction, means that very soon you feel worse than you did before you started taking the drug – even when you are actually taking it and experiencing the 'high', you feel worse than you would had you never taken it. The same is true of eating badly. You may eat something bad for you that you have trained yourself to enjoy, and you may obtain some pleasure from it at the time, but the health problems it causes, which slowly increase over time, make you feel worse off overall.

It is easiest to visualise this using a simple diagram. Look at the chart below. The figures on the vertical line on the left represent happiness, with nil being neither happy nor sad, and increasing numbers being happier and decreasing numbers being sadder. The horizontal line at the bottom represents time passing. Each time you eat something bad for you, or take a drug (like alcohol, caffeine or nicotine), you get a small, momentary boost. But over time, as the effect of the drug or the effect of constantly eating unhealthy food takes effect, we feel worse off generally. As you can see, we do get a boost each time we eat or take the drug, but we very quickly become far worse off overall.

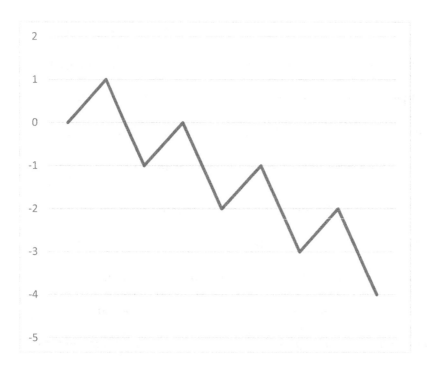

This is one of the key points to bear in mind. You cannot feel better than having a fit body and the resilient, healthy mind that goes with it. No drug or food can give you this feeling. It can take it away, and then partially restore it, but any benefit it confers is an illusion.

Healthy living is not about living longer or looking good (although both of these are direct results of healthy living); it is about enjoying life to the full.

Eating to relieve stress doesn't work. Hunger is a form of stress, and eating will relieve it, so your subconscious starts to associate eating with relief of stress. This is compounded by the dopamine element, and is further compounded by the refined sugar rush. However, overeating and eating the wrong type of food just compounds the problem. Poor diet leads to reduced health, which in turn leads to mental fragility and an increasingly emotive state, causing an ever increasing desire to keep eating rubbish.

Do you tend to eat when you are not hungry if you are bored and miserable? Is there this same tendency when you are excited and happy? Do you think being fat and lethargic is more or less likely to make you feel bored and miserable? In this way overeating is a vicious circle, a very frustrating and unrewarding one. Just remember you can get a temporary, small and guilt-laden 'boost' from eating, or a genuine, day-long beneficial boost from doing a bit of exercise.

Exercise and the long-term boost you get from eating properly don't dull your emotions, they make you feel like you can deal with whatever life throws at you. They allow you to see the comedy in life, to not let things grind you down.

If you haven't exercised before, or haven't exercised for some time, the first few sessions will be difficult, not only in terms of the exercise but also in terms of how self-conscious you will feel. If you do feel very self-conscious, then think on this: how many joggers have you seen in your life? And how many would you actually recognise if they came up to you right now? I bet not a single one, unless you see the same one on a very regular basis. How many walkers or cyclists have you seen in your life? Again, how many could you actually identify? Isn't it the case that you see so many of them that you scarcely even notice them anymore? If you are in your tracksuit, hovering by the front door trying to pluck up enough courage to actually leave the house, remember that the chances are that not one single person you see will even consciously register your existence, and even if they do you'll be almost instantly forgotten. The first time is the worst. It gets progressively easier and even (and I'm afraid you will just have to trust me on this!) more enjoyable every time you go out.

Whilst this book is not about telling you what to do (it is about giving you information and helping you see things in a different way, about encouraging to you to use your own experiences and apply your own judgement, and about letting you put it to what use you will), I think it is useful for illustrative purposes just to give you a snapshot of my life. Firstly, it shows you how forgiving the whole process is, and secondly, how quick and easy meals can be. One of the problem with eating unprocessed food is you could end up having to go to the shops every day to get fresh food, and preparing meals from scratch can take ages. For most people this just isn't practical.

The first thing I do every day is have a cup of coffee or tea (see how I am already deviating from the ideal?). A couple of times a week I will go for a run in the morning. I also put some fruit and fresh veg (and sometimes a pinch of salt) in a blender and make a smoothie to take to work. It takes five minutes. We get our shopping weekly. Towards the beginning of the week the fruit and veg that goes in is fresh, towards the end of the week I use frozen. My smoothie, along with a big bag of nuts, goes to work with me. I usually have more tea during the morning, head to the gym for 20 minutes or so at lunchtime, have my smoothie when I get back to my desk, then have the nuts later in the afternoon. When I get home I'll have a salad with nuts or fish, and often whatever is left over from my boys' dinner (pasta, pizza, whatever). Again the salad is for earlier in the week, then later in the week I'll often put a pack of microwave rice, frozen veg, and a tin of lentils of chickpeas in a saucepan and heat it all up, then flavour it with soy sauce or a curry sauce or something. Five minutes packet to plate. I used to spend all evening eating, but now I make sure I don't eat anything after dinner. Weekends I stray even further. I choose fresh fruit and vegetables if I can, but often if we are out for children's parties or meals out, I just have to choose the best I can.

Can you see how easy and forgiving it is? How far from the ideal I am, yet how it still works? How I apply the principles is largely dictated by my circumstances – I'd love to give up caffeine but with a young family and a full time job I never seem to get enough sleep as it is. My job pays me a good wage to use my brain, but I cannot do my job on five hours' sleep and no caffeine. Sometimes we scarcely seem to get any sleep at all, yet every day I have to be in that office, mentally firing on all cylinders. Also,

I would quite happily eat fresh food for every meal, but I simply don't have the time to firstly shop for it, then to prepare it. I am not vegan, or even vegetarian, but I am probably 90% vegan, and 95% vegetarian. Again, this is dictated more from circumstances and practicalities than choice. For me this particular issue is about far more than health and fitness, it is about animal welfare, about treating other creatures with dignity and kindness, about negotiating this maze of a life that we are all trying to find our way through without causing needless pain and suffering to other living things. In nature many, many animals eat other animals. But I am not concerned about this, I am only concerned about what I do, about taking what steps I personally can. There is a story about a person who is walking along the beach, the tide is going out and there are thousands upon thousands of star fish all washing up on the beach dying, stretching for miles and miles. They then see someone else on the beach who is picking up starfish and throwing them back. They say to them, 'What on earth are you doing? There are thousands of washed up starfish. How can you possible make a difference?' The person picks up a starfish, throws it into the sea and says, 'Well I made a difference to that one.' For me it is about doing what you can, no matter how insignificant it might seem. However, this is my personal choice and such moral considerations are for each individual to decide for themselves.

Let me be quite clear. Although the regime is forgiving, you shouldn't treat it as 70% or whatever fruit and veg, then 30% what you 'do enjoy'. If you do this you just place yourself on a permanent diet, i.e. you restrict food rather than alter what you genuinely want to eat. This is about changing your eating habits, not restricting what you eat. You should be aware of how forgiving it is not so you can abuse it, but so that in situations where your choice is genuinely limited, you can make the best choice from what is available without thinking you've blown it, or even if you just really fancy something, you can have it without worrying. This is a subtle point but an important one. The flexibility should allow you to deviate in unusual circumstances, or when practicalities dictate.

The flexibility also allows you to be sensible and find a compromise between a natural diet and modern living. Our natural diet is best suited for 'natural living', but most of us don't live 'natural lives'. For example, when humans move around their oxygen intake increases and adrenaline is released so we are kept awake. If we sit down for any length of time our body thinks it is a rest period, and takes the opportunity to send us off to sleep. That would be fine if we were still living in the wilderness, but we aren't. I do an office job. I am sat down for 8 to 10 hours a day, either reading, writing or talking. Even when I had given up caffeine for some considerable period, so was well and truly over the physical withdrawal, and even when I had slept well, I still struggled getting through the day without tea or coffee because I would end up nodding off. Of course the ideal would be to pop out every few hours for a quick run or brisk walk to wake up, but how many of us have the time to do that? Equally, if you decide you want to run an ultramarathon you probably aren't going to get your best time eating fruit and vegetables.

You need to find the right balance that suits you. The purpose of this book is not to dictate what you should or shouldn't do, it is to help you understand the whole diet and fitness phenomenon, to give you information so you can make your own decisions, to make you think about what you eat and why, and make sure you are happy you are doing the right thing for you.

We've already dealt with how to move towards a better diet and fitness routine, but I think it is worth going over it again in this conclusion. The main parts, when you actually get down to basics, are actually small in number, and can be broken down into eight points.

1.  You are not going to eat every time you are 'hungry'. You are going to be drilling down to see which aspects of hunger are involved and striving to only eat when you are genuinely hungry (i.e. there is a lack of nutrients and/or energy).

2.  The food you will be eating more of will taste different to what you are used to. It won't taste worse, in fact it will taste significantly better, but it is different.

3.  Thirdly, and perhaps more importantly that the taste, it will have a different texture. It is a different experience eating it. Without a thorough analysis you might almost describe the new food as being a 'less satisfying' eating experience.

Chewing an apple isn't as 'satisfying' as eating a big mouthful of chocolate or pizza or burger. But when you analyse it further you realise that, over time and with years of bad diet, you have come to associate the bloating that comes from eating processed food (which is actually the feeling you get when you eat something that your body is not designed to digest and therefore will struggle to process) with being 'full' or 'satisfied'. It is not actually a satisfying texture, but a texture that tells you that you are eating something that will make you feel bloated and lethargic.

4. Leading on from this (and this is connected to the previous point but I think it is useful to separate it out and treat it separately), your new diet won't leave you feeling bloated. Because you have spent so many years associating this feeling of bloating with satisfying your hunger, it will feel odd when you don't feel it. You will be hungry, you will eat, you will stop feeling hungry, you will stop eating. You are going to stop eating when you get even the merest indication you are

starting to get full. The rest of the food goes in the fridge for another meal, or in the bin. When you eat there will be no accompanying feeling of bloating. This will feel strange to begin with as you can misunderstand this and it can feel like you should be eating more. Soon you will stop associating this physical feeling of distended organs with being 'satisfied', and you will no longer seek it out every time you eat. This bloated feeling is both a cause and a symptom of poor eating habits. Just remember that the feeling is neither a good nor a natural feeling, it is something you will be very glad to see that back of. The only reason you have eaten to this level for so many years is because that is all you've known and you have misunderstood what that feeling actually signifies.

5.   You are going to be beating your cravings rather than giving in to them. The more you do this, the easier it gets, and as you get used to your new diet you will start to crave healthy food, rather than unhealthy food, so you will no longer need to give in to them anyway. And as you stop reaching for the

food every time you have a setback, so your subconscious will start to learn new rules and those subconscious triggers will dwindle and die.

6. You will be eating slowly and deliberately. This may sound easy, but it will take some work, particularly as you are now going to be eating only when you are genuinely hungry, which tends to increase the desire to eat quickly.

7. That is it as far as diet goes. The only other change is the exercise point. If you are someone who doesn't exercise at the moment you are probably looking at about 20 minutes, three times a week, to begin with. It may feel strange to start, but you only need to spend a total of one hour a week exercising; that is one hour out of 168. The one hour will leave you feeling immeasurably better, help you sleep better, and in no time at all will be the highlight of your day.

8. The final point only applies to those giving up a drug as part of their new regime. Stopping drinking, smoking, consuming caffeine, etc. is outside the scope of this book and I don't intend covering it in detail, but you should be aware that there will be a short physical adjustment/withdrawal period while your brain adjusts to having a drug withdrawn that it has grown used to having forced on it on a regular basis, usually for some years. The physical side effects of this usually last no more than five days. If you do want to understand drug addiction, then this is covered in more detail in *Alcohol Explained.*

The thing you will notice about all of these points is that the effort is at the start, then it gets progressively easier and soon it will be natural and require no effort at all. So as the new becomes the norm, and as you start to really see the benefits of your new life, so it will start to take on a life of its own. There really is no comparison between the two lives, your new life and your old one, and you will start to see the benefits almost immediately, but the beauty is that you continue to improve for months on end. And when I talk about improvement I am not talking about losing weight and looking slimmer, I am talking about the confidence and energy and mental resilience that come from having a healthy body that isn't under constant stress from poor diet. Believe it or not, the weight loss and change of body shape is nothing compared to the huge improvement to your quality of life. It is a very pleasant side effect, but far from the main benefit.

If you have found this book useful, then I would ask two things of you. Firstly, please leave a review on Amazon, which is this book's main marketing platform. Secondly, please recommend it. Whether a book is recommended by those who read it ultimately dictates whether it lives or dies.

Finally, if you would like to join the Diet and Fitness Explained community, I have set up a Facebook Group called (rather predictably) 'Diet and Fitness Explained'. I hope to see you there.